A-HARROWI.. ..
We Shall Go

Exploring the Harrow Way:
Britain's 'Oldest Road'

Annabel Stowe

Printed by Mayfield Press (Oxford) Limited, 2021
Unit 4, Ashville Way, Oxford OX4 6TU

Romanroving@gmail.com

The Historical and Archaeological Notes for each walk are based to a
large extent on data from the Hampshire Historic Environment Record
(HER), kindly provided by Alan Whitney, Historic Data Manager,
Hampshire County Council. Helpful information was also provided by
David Hopkins, Hampshire County Archaeologist, HCC.

Routes and information are accurate at the time of going to press.
The author cannot be held responsible for any subsequent changes.
She has taken all reasonable steps to ensure that these walks are safe.
However, all outdoor activities involve an element of risk, and she can
accept no responsibility for any injuries caused to readers following
these walks.

ISBN 978-1-3999-0279-3

The Harrow Way through the Ages

Eight circular walks across
North-West Hampshire
between
Oakley and Cholderton
trace this ancient
trackway's long history

This Walking Guide takes you on a journey with 'Harrow Wayfarers' down through the millennia. Each walk focuses on a different historical period.

It is based on thorough research, with a pinch of imaginative licence to bring the past alive.

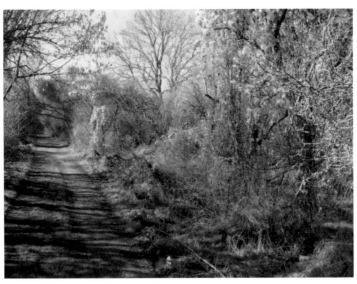

The Harrow Way north of Overton, in late winter

Very old are we men;
Our dreams are tales
Told in dim Eden
By Eve's nightingales;
We wake and whisper awhile,
But, the day gone by,
Silence and sleep like fields
Of amaranth lie.

from *All That's Past**
Walter de la Mare
1873-1956

In memory of Marija,
our 'digging' friend

*by kind permission of The Society of Authors, as representatives of
The Literary Trustees of Walter de la Mare

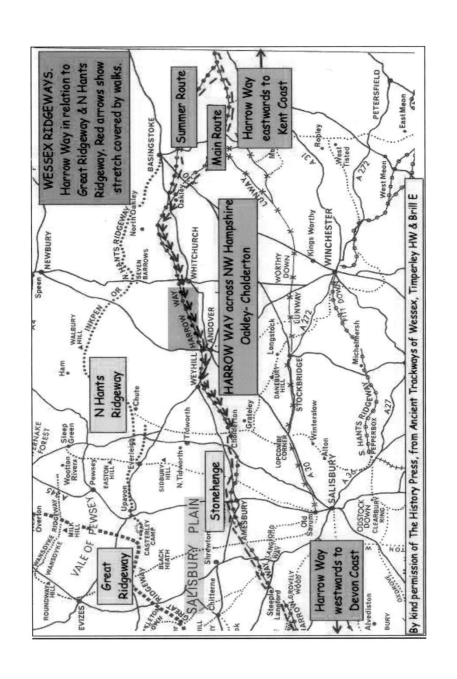

WESSEX RIDGEWAYS. Harrow Way in relation to Great Ridgeway & N Hants Ridgeway. Red arrows show stretch covered by walks.

Summer Route

Main Route

Harrow Way eastwards to Kent Coast

N Hants Ridgeway

HARROW WAY across NW Hampshire Oakley- Cholderton

Great Ridgeway

Stonehenge

Harrow Way westwards to Devon Coast

By kind permission of The History Press, from Ancient Trackways of Wessex, Timperley HW & Brill E

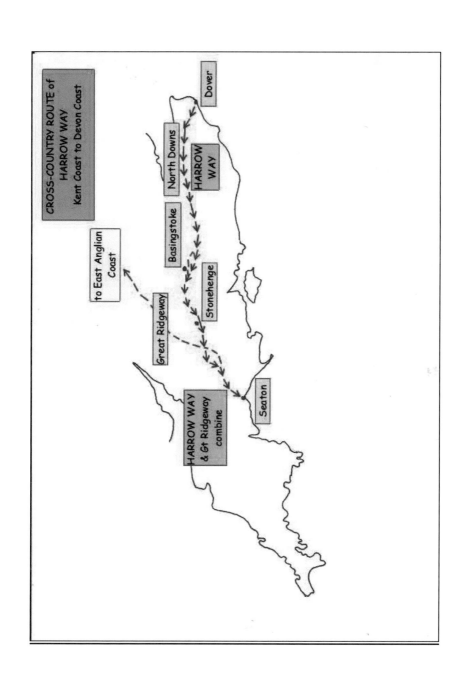

CROSS-COUNTRY ROUTE of HARROW WAY
Kent Coast to Devon Coast

Dover

North Downs

HARROW WAY

Basingstoke

Stonehenge

Great Ridgeway

to East Anglian Coast

HARROW WAY & Gt Ridgeway combine

Seaton

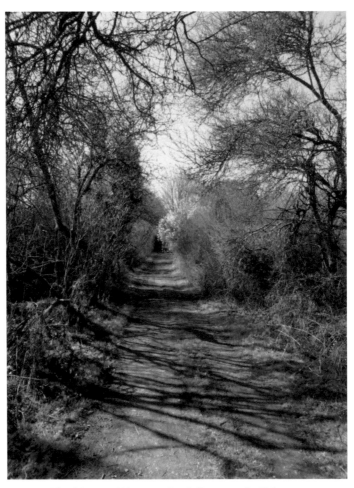

The Harrow Way north of Overton, in February

CONTENTS

INTRODUCTION

Circular walks from the Harrow Way/Harroway

This Guide contains eight circular walks, ranging from approx 7km/4.3miles to 14km/8.7miles, incorporating the best-preserved or most accessible stretches of the Harrow Way across NW Hampshire, from Oakley in the east to Cholderton in the west, on the Wiltshire border. They explore some of the prettiest countryside in the county – the green lane running to the north of Overton and Whitchurch is particularly unspoilt, and makes for glorious walking, (especially between November and May, when it is closed to off-road vehicles).

Snapshots in time, in historical sequence

The walks are not intended to be strung together on a point-to-point basis along the Harrow Way – too much has been lost or lies under busy modern roads – but rather as a series of snapshots in time, each focusing on a different period, from Palaeolithic/Mesolithic through to Post-Medieval. Walks are therefore arranged in historical, rather than geographical, sequence, starting with the oldest, to give the feeling of walking the 'Harrow Way through the Ages'. Although this prehistoric trackway may not have extended right across the country until the Bronze Age, local tracks justify the inclusion here of walks from earlier periods.

1

'Harrow Wayfarers'

Each walk follows in the footsteps of imaginary 'Harrow Wayfarers' - a term coined by the author to describe those who might have been using the trackway in each period - to help bring the past alive and give today's rambler some engaging company!

A Linear Walk

The last walk (approx 13km/8.1miles) along the Harrow Way is linear, taking in the green lane between Overton and Whitchurch, with start/end points accessible by public transport. It has a slightly different focus to the circular walks, and is intended as a fitting conclusion to the 'Harrow Way Experience'.

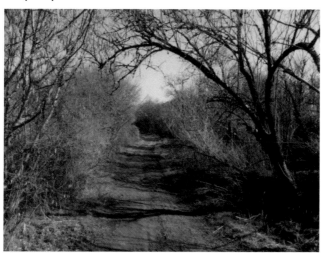

The Harrow Way, a green lane, north of Overton

PREHISTORIC RIDGEWAYS

From high ways to highways

As traffic thunders west along the A303 out of Basingstoke, heading, perhaps, for the delights of Devon or Cornwall, uppermost in drivers' minds - in these pre-tunnel days - is the hope that there will be no hold-up round Stonehenge. Few, indeed probably none at all, will be reflecting that the origins of this highway lie way back in prehistory, when the main thoroughfares were, quite literally, 'high ways' running along the chalk ridges forming the backbone of Southern England.

High and dry

For millennia after the end of the last Ice Age, around 10,000 years ago, valley floors were treacherous, inhospitable places. Wolves and wild boar hunted in the deciduous woodland that had sprung up as the climate warmed. Riverside bogs would ensnare the unsuspecting traveller, or at least impede his progress. Far better to follow the drier ground of the ridges, to reach the next habitation, or take animals to watering holes. So these watershed ways linked hilltops, descending as little as possible to the lower ground.

The 'Oldest Roads in Britain'

For several thousand years, then, these ancient high ways formed a vital infrastructure across the South of England, fanning outwards from the central plateau of Salisbury Plain, following the ridges to, ultimately, the coast. Although they were not created as long-distance, continuous routes, but as local tracks, in time short stretches linked up to form a more extensive network. The two most ancient ridgeways that vie for the title 'Oldest Road in Britain', namely the **Great Ridgeway** and the **Harrow Way,** ran roughly east-west across the country, from the present day East Anglian coast, in the case of the former, and East Kent for the latter. Both reached the sea again at the chalk cliffs of South Devon. (See map *Wessex Ridgeways* in frontispieces).

How old are these 'Oldest Roads'?

Did the **Great Ridgeway** exist before Britain became an island (broadly speaking cBC6000), as has been claimed by some, or is this an over-exaggeration of its antiquity? The **Harrow Way** is believed to date from at least the Bronze Age (BC2200-801), as we shall see. But what is the evidence *on the ground?* Interestingly, in places the Harrow Way appears to have a relationship with the 'Celtic' field systems (see *Glossary*) to the north, suggesting it may have been contemporary with, or even predated, these, which can date from any time from the Early Bronze Age (BC2200-1601) onwards (*Footnote i*). And the Harrow Way pre-Bronze Age? The abundance of finds from earlier periods suggests, to the author at least, the passage of still older travellers.

Footnote i: observations of historic landscape character by the Hampshire County Archaeologist.

ORIGINS of the HARROW WAY

A valuable commodity

So why did the Harrow Way become such an important thoroughfare in the Bronze Age? One of the answers lies in Cornwall. TIN. When mixed with copper, this makes a stronger, more durable metal than copper alone. BRONZE. And tin was relatively rare, at least major deposits were. For the flourishing civilisations of the Eastern Mediterranean (Egyptian, Mycenaean and Canaanite, amongst others), copper was found 'on the spot', in Cyprus (the clue is in the name), but tin had to be sourced further afield. So people had to be prepared to travel great distances, or at least have access to trade routes, along which commodities could change hands, in order to get hold of the raw materials they required.

Cornwall-bound along the Harrow Way

An overland route from the Eastern Mediterranean may have brought traders and metalworkers into Britain on the coast of Kent, at the shortest sea crossing, then along the chalk ridges westwards, as we shall see shortly. One maritime route may have come up the western seaboard of Europe, past the Iberian Peninsula and France, to make landfall in Christchurch Bay, before heading north along tracks to join the Harrow Way, then on to the West Country.

Stonehenge-bound along the Harrow Way

Both of the above journeys would have led past the ceremonial centres of Salisbury Plain, a numinous landscape long before the Bronze Age, and this may offer a further explanation for the importance of the Harrow Way. Both these strands (the route to Cornwall's tin, the route to Stonehenge) seem to come together in one person – the so-called 'Amesbury Archer' (now in The Salisbury Museum) buried near Stonehenge, close to the Harrow Way, around BC2300. Isotope analysis of his teeth shows origins in the Alpine region, so had he, as has been suggested, travelled over a thousand miles in search of pain relief (he had no left kneecap) through the healing properties of the bluestones at Stonehenge, re-positioned around this time? Or was he, perhaps, an incomer bringing new metalworking skills, as his copious grave goods included delicately-wrought hair braids (the first gold found in Britain), and cushion stones, used as portable anvils, suggesting he may have been a coppersmith? We can only surmise what brought him here, and how he made the long journey, but he does seem to epitomise the key role played by the Harrow Way, in leading both to the source of tin and to Stonehenge.

So our Harrow Way may have been in its prime in the Bronze Age. But was that the end of the story? Read on …

HARROW WAY: TRACKWAY through the AGES

As we have just seen, this ancient track probably goes back at least as far as the Bronze Age (BC2200-801), when it extended right across Southern England, coast to coast. Before we consider the successive incarnations of the Harrow Way, and the route it took, let's look at its name.

What's in a name? Well rather a lot, actually
Hoare or *har-* denote 'ancient', as in 'hoary'. The first reference to the 'Hoare Way' is in an Anglo-Saxon charter of around AD900. Generic terms for a ridgeway or watershed way include *hryceweg*, *hereweg* ('army way' or 'through road') and *Weale-weg*, meaning 'Welsh way', as the Anglo-Saxons used the term 'Welsh' to refer to the indigenous British tribes they had conquered. 'Welsh way' was also a term used for a drove road.

Phew! Let's pause a moment to take all that in.

'Way to the shrine'
To this bewildering array of Old English names, *hearg weg* can be added. Meaning 'way to the shrine or holy place', it could well refer to Stonehenge. Alternatively, or additionally, it could be a reference to the shrine of St Swithun, as a branch track led from the Harrow Way southwards to Winchester. But Swithun was not the only saint to draw pilgrims along the Harrow Way. The route from Farnham to Canterbury is still known as the

Pilgrims' Way, being the route followed by Medieval pilgrims to the shrine of Archbishop Thomas Becket, after his murder in AD1170 at the hands of his erstwhile friend, King Henry II.

Route of the Harrow Way
(see maps in frontispieces)
The reader not over-familiar with this area may be starting to ask, but where exactly is it? What is its route? Residents of Andover or Basingstoke will know it as a school or a road respectively, but clearly there is more to it than that! In a nutshell, the Harrow Way runs east to west, starting near the White Cliffs of Dover, running along the chalk ridge of the North Downs, past Guildford and Farnham, to enter Hampshire. Just east of Long Sutton, sources suggest that the route forks: the main, more southerly, route going through Ellisfield and Farleigh Wallop, whilst the more northerly section – possibly used in the summer – passes just south of Basingstoke. They re-join at Oakley, west of Basingstoke. Continuing on its westerly journey, the Harrow Way runs to the north of Overton and Whitchurch (roughly parallel to the Portway Roman Road from Silchester to Old Sarum) before passing Andover, Weyhill and on to Amesbury and Stonehenge. The exact line of the Harrow Way west of Weyhill is the subject of debate, but this Guide uses the route described by Timperley and Brill in *Ancient Trackways of Wessex* (see *References and Sources* p156) running between Quarley Hill and Cholderton Hill, rather than to

8

the north of the latter. On the chalk downs of Wiltshire, having passed close to Stonehenge, the Harrow Way joins the other contender for the title 'Oldest Road in Britain', the Great Ridgeway, coming from its point of entry on the coast of East Anglia. Together they cross Somerset, where it is difficult to distinguish one from the other, and on into Devon, terminating on the coast near the chalk cliffs of Beer and Seaton, at the mouth of the River Axe - from the White Cliffs of Dover in the east to the White Cliffs of Beer in the west.

A trackway through the ages
From its probable prehistoric origins, the Harrow Way continued in use for hundreds of years until the arrival of the Romans on our shores in AD43. Although evidence is scarce, especially in the area covered by this Guide, of these enthusiastic road-builders commandeering the Harrow Way for their own ends, it was clearly still a busy *weg* in the Early Medieval period (AD410-1065), after the withdrawal of Roman administration in AD410. In this period too it served to demarcate land boundaries, the forerunners of our parish boundaries. In its different guises as drove road, trackway, watershed way, trade route, thoroughfare, pilgrims' way and ridgeway, it rolled on through the Middle Ages (AD1066-1539) and Post-Medieval period (1540-1900) into the 18th and 19th centuries, when stretches became the new

turnpike roads. But that was not the end of it. Even today, the A303, overlying parts of the Harrow Way, as we have seen, still bears motorists westwards towards Salisbury Plain – holidaymakers replacing the pilgrims and shepherds of old – and the parts that have escaped tarmac-isation (new word) still present the rambler with pleasant green lanes, tracks and footpaths, as we shall see.

So the Harrow Way has had a long and varied history, and, though fragmented, is still there to be discovered and enjoyed.

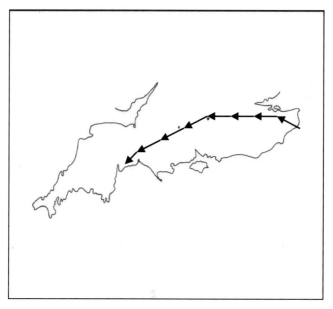

Approximate coast-to-coast route of the Harrow Way

TIME PERIODS and WALKS INDEX

TIME PERIOD	DATES	WALK (blue shading =best for Harroway)	PAGE
Palaeolithic	BC500,000-10001	1)ST MARY BOURNE 8.2km/5.1miles Easy/Moderate	15
Mesolithic	BC10000-4001		
Neolithic	BC4000-2201	2)NUTBANE 8.5km/5.3miles Easy/Moderate	29
Bronze Age	BC2200-801	3)OVERTON 14km/8.7miles Challenging	47
Iron Age	BC800-AD42	4)QUARLEY HILL 7km/4.3miles Easy	63
Roman	AD43-409	5)CHOLDERTON 12km/7.5miles Moderate	77
Early Medieval / Anglo-Saxon	AD410-1065	6)WHITCHURCH 11km/6.8miles Moderate	91
Medieval	AD1066-1539	7)DEANE 12km/7.5miles Moderate	111
Post-Medieval	AD1540-1900	8)OVERTON & Ashe 10.5km/6.5miles Moderate	129
LINEAR WALK: A FINAL HARROW WAY EXPERIENCE 13km/8.1miles Challenging p 145			

11

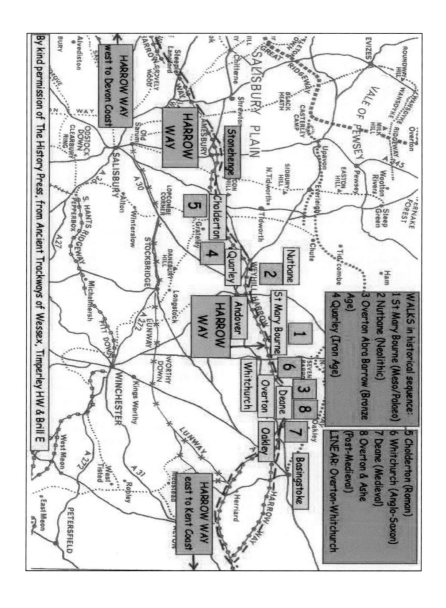

GUIDELINES for walks:

>The Practical Information box at the start of each walk gives useful details.

>**OS Explorer maps 131 (Romsey, Andover & Test Valley) and 144 (Basingstoke, Alton & Whitchurch) are needed, to supplement the simple maps in the text.**

>On the route maps, directions are in yellow boxes, historical and archaeological features in red boxes, with corresponding notes and a timeline after the route description.

>Remember to follow the Country Code, including taking litter home and keeping dogs under control.

>Walks are undertaken at your own risk. Take **great care** when walking near, or crossing, busy roads. High visibility waistcoats are recommended.

>Walking poles may be helpful, in places.

>Note that the Harrow Way is closed to off-road vehicles November-March, but scrambling bikes are allowed at all times of year.

>Please note that ancient monuments are usually on private land, but viewable from a right of way.

>Each walk indicates the Harrow Way in blue.

>Each walk has a pub/tea room on route or nearby.

>Visits to local museums strongly recommended. Note that displays may change from time to time.

>Visit websites for all opening times, and bus/train timetables.

GUIDE to GRADES based on distance & terrain:

EASY = up to approx 8km/5miles

MODERATE = up to approx 13km/8.1miles

CHALLENGING = over 13km/8.1miles

WALKS and their HARROW WAYFARERS

WALK 1: Setting the Scene
HARROW WAYFARERS in the MESOLITHIC (BC10000-4001) and
Palaeolithic (BC500,000-10001)

Mesolithic (Middle Stone Age) **Man** favoured the dry chalk ridges for travel, and the valley floors for his seasonal camps, where the wooded areas provided him with dinner. Though by now the game was less impressively huge than the woolly mammoths of the Palaeolithic (a giant tusk on display in the Willis Museum gives an idea of scale – see photo p163) and less savage than the sabre-toothed tigers, it was still plentiful and tasty. Wild boar, wolves, deer, wild oxen, and smaller mammals such as foxes and pine martens could be hunted with tools fashioned from flint or bone, and fish, along with nuts and berries, would contribute to a healthier diet than ours in the 21stcentury.

On the shores of swampy, reed-fringed lakes, or on dry mounds and hillocks above the marshy hollows, he constructed simple shelters, and began to manage his environment. Woodland clearance was starting, for Mesolithic Man realised that small open spaces among the oak, elm, ash, hazel and alder would encourage deer and wild cattle to graze, making them easier targets. Doubtless the numerous tranchet axes (see *Glossary*) found in Hampshire – and on the site of this walk – were put to good use. But was Mesolithic Man using the Harrow Way? As we have seen, it may only have been a local track at this time, but he was

15

certainly close to it. Ground-breaking excavations in recent years at Blick Mead, Amesbury, are revealing a settlement spanning several thousand years, from cBC9600 to cBC4000. Algae in the spring water turn flints a rich pink, as magical to the eye of the modern beholder as, surely, to his prehistoric ancestors. (A visit to Amesbury History Centre is recommended).

And what of **Palaeolithic** (Old Stone Age) **Man**, back in the mists of prehistory? Time, and the movement of ice sheets, have obliterated his tracks, but someone dropped, discarded or deposited two handaxes here in the Bourne Valley, half a million years ago ...

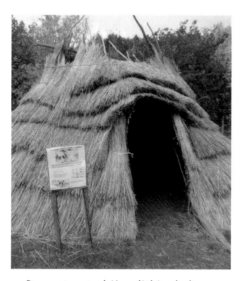

Reconstructed Mesolithic shelter,
courtesy of Butser Ancient Farm

WALK 1 ROUTE MAP (OS Explorer 144 or 131)

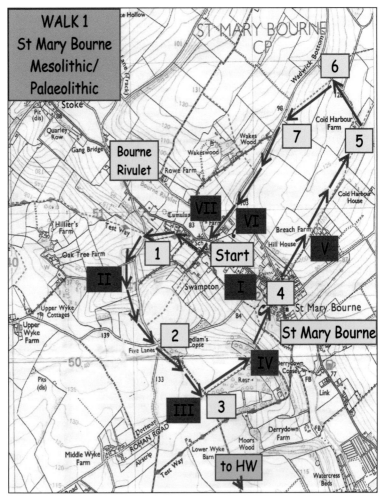

© Crown copyright and database rights 2021 OS Licence 100059949

WALK 1: ST MARY BOURNE
Focus on the MESOLITHIC (BC10000-4001) & Palaeolithic (BC500,000-10001)

From prehistoric trackway to sleepy, stream-side village and windswept down-land

As the stretch of the Harrow Way for this walk would be along a busy road, it links instead with a branch track, running S-N, crossing the Harrow Way just west of Chapman's Ford, before heading northwards along the western ridge of the Bourne Valley to join, ultimately, the North Hampshire Ridgeway (see map p27). Both Mesolithic and Palaeolithic Man have left ample evidence of their passage in the Bourne Valley.

Practical Information:
Distance:approx **8.2km/5.1miles. Easy/Moderate**
Parking: On road at the northern end of St Mary Bourne, near the school. Please park sensitively.
Refreshments/Toilets: George Inn in the village centre, on the walk. The Bourne Inn is a short distance down the valley. No public toilets.
Terrain: Undulating, with some steep-ish ascents and descents. Footpaths (may be muddy), tracks and quiet country lanes. Three stiles with dog gates. Dogs on lead where indicated. Take care on/crossing roads.
Map:OS Explorer 144 (also 131).
Grid ref at start point:SU416 507
Best time of year: Any clear day, though not after prolonged rain. Breezy sunshine in spring, perhaps, with primroses and violets in the hedgerows.

18

About the Walk:

Climbing from the sheltered village to exposed ridges and open down-land, along footpaths, tracks and country lanes (Test Way and Brenda Parker Way - visit websites), this exhilarating walk links with a prehistoric branch track of the Harrow Way, takes in a Roman road, and passes close to significant prehistoric and Roman findspots. A dry walk in hot weather, but the flood plain, after prolonged rain, shows the rambler why Mesolithic Man preferred to avoid the marshy valley floor!

Highlights from the Mesolithic/Palaeolithic:

Abundant finds, including:
>Mesolithic:19 tranchet axes, 6 blade cores, 2 blades and flakes, and a pick
>Palaeolithic:2 handaxes and 8 flint implements
Highlights from other periods:
>Roman road and Roman pottery findspots
>Neolithic polished axe (fragment) findspot
>Medieval church

Imagine the Scene in the Mesolithic:

Down in the valley, on a dry mound surrounded by swampy hollows, a group of hunter-gatherers is making preparations for an expedition. Leaving their kinsmen to hunt deer in the wildwood, process antlers, tan hides, fish or forage, they plan to head up to a ridgeway above the valley that will take them southwards to join the Harrow Way. They have heard of a spring in the west with magical properties ...

19

At the northern end of the long village of St Mary Bourne (I) roadside parking should be possible near the school and the Coronation Arms (sadly vacant at the time of writing). Please park sensitively.

START: Between the Coronation Arms and the school, walk down **School Lane**. Follow the lane along by the school, round the corner to the **RIGHT** for approx **30m**, then leave the lane to fork **LEFT** up a track. Just beyond 'Nutwood', turn **RIGHT** along the **Test Way,** to follow a narrow path (may be muddy) between hedge and fence. Keep straight on, towards an attractive barn conversion with a half-hipped roof, and possibly geese in the garden, past a line of trees in the middle of a field on your left, perhaps marking an old boundary. The village is soon left behind as you make your way along by fields and meadows. Go through a metal gate and follow the **Test Way** diagonally **LEFT** up the slope, (mind the electric fence), along a grassy track at the right edge of the field. At the top of the slope, go through the metal gate, then turn immediately **RIGHT** through a wooded area. After approx **100m** you pass through another metal gate onto a very quiet country lane. Leave the **Test Way** here and turn **LEFT** to follow the lane.

(1) This quiet country lane is the **prehistoric branch track of the Harrow Way (II)** (see map p27). It undulates over down-land, with views of

20

the Bourne Valley to the left, where the Bourne Rivulet flows at the foot of the far slope, and isolated thatched cottages add charm to the rural scene.   As you set off southwards along this ancient route, you might like to imagine the Mesolithic hunter-gatherers, setting off towards the **Harrow Way**, having climbed up from their camp in the valley (see 'Imagine the Scene').   Go down the hill into the dip, and take the **LEFT** fork. There may be a short stretch of flooding here, after prolonged rain, but it should be possible to get along the verge. A long-ish, steep-ish climb follows (donkeys, perhaps, on the left). Avoid the temptation to follow one of the numerous footpaths over fields, and carry on to the ancient **meeting of five lanes**, marked on the OS map.

(2) At this crossroads, go **STRAIGHT AHEAD** along a tarmac lane - a public footpath, cycle route 246, and part of the Brenda Parker Way (visit website) – passing between farm buildings, until you come to a thick conifer hedge on the right. Keep to the right of a Nissen hut, to emerge onto an open field with a track leading straight ahead. This is exposed country, with big skies and wide horizons. Continue **STRAIGHT ACROSS** the field to the far hedge. Here you leave the Harrow Wayfarers to continue their journey to the **Harrow Way**, which lies approx 1.4km ahead. At the corner of the hedge, pause to look right and left, and you will see a clear straight path – this is the Portway Roman Road (III) (see Walk 5).

(3) At the corner of the hedge, turn **LEFT** onto the Portway, following a path along the right edge of the field, with the hedge on your right. At the end of the field, follow the path into the trees, bearing diagonally left between coppiced beeches. On your right at this point, on private land, are important Stone Age and Roman findspots (IV). A short, steep descent follows, to bring you to a grassy track, leading down to **St Mary Bourne Lake**, in the SE corner of which more Roman Pottery (IV) was found, when the lake was created. At the foot of the slope, go **LEFT** through the metal gate into the Sports Field then bear **RIGHT** to follow the right edge of the field, along by a line of trees that fringes the lake, where wild geese, ducks and waterfowl enjoy the watery expanse. Leave the Sports Field by the village shop – conveniently placed right by the path. Go **STRAIGHT AHEAD** to the main village road, and almost opposite is the equally conveniently-placed **George Inn**, where some refreshment might be needed, at roughly the mid-point of the walk. Before continuing, a visit to the nearby Church of St Peter, with its relatively-rare 12[th]century Tournai marble font, is recommended.

(4) Return to the George Inn, and look for **Spring Hill Lane** leading off to the **left** when you are facing the pub. Follow Spring Hill Lane for a short distance. Just as it begins to climb, watch for a **steep drive** on the right, and just to the **right** of this, almost hidden in the hedge, a **footpath sign**.

Go up the steps and along the narrow, sheltered path as it climbs, shortly coming to a track. Follow this uphill, past a **Woodland Burial Ground** on the left. Over to the right in Breach Field, on private land, extensive scatters of Stone Age tools and implements (V) were found. When the track you are on makes a sharp bend to the **right,** just past the new-build houses on the right, **leave the track** to continue **STRAIGHT AHEAD** along a **grassy footpath** at the right edge of the field, with a line of conifers on your right giving welcome shelter from easterly winds. At the end of the field, cross a **stile with dog gate**, then across a further **two** fields with stiles (and possibly woolly occupants – dogs on lead), until you emerge onto a quiet country lane by **Cold Harbour Farm,** an attractive 19[th]century building, with a patch of hellebores in season creating a colourful picture in the corner of the garden.

(5) At Cold Harbour Farm, bear **LEFT** along the lane, gradually cresting the ridge, before beginning the long descent towards **Wadwick Bottom**. This is wonderful upland country, with views opening up to the north now.

(6) Approx **150m before the white signpost** in the valley bottom, watch for a **solitary oak** on the right, shortly followed by a **gap** in the hedge on the **left** (may be overgrown, and the sign difficult to spot). Leave the lane here to turn **LEFT** into a field. If there is a clear strip path cut through the crop, heading **diagonally** across the field, take this, otherwise follow the perimeter of the field along the top edge, then round to the right and down the slope to the road. (If you miss the gap in the hedge to bring you into this field, simply continue down the road to **Wadwick Bottom** and turn left).

(7) When you reach Wadwick Bottom, turn **LEFT**, and follow the road back south-westwards towards St Mary Bourne. After approx **1km**, as you begin the descent down Baptist Hill, with a pleasant view of the village and river in the valley, there is a findspot **(VI)** on the left. The road brings you down over the bridge and back into the village, opposite School Lane, where the walk began. Before returning to the car, walk a few metres to the right, towards the picturesque thatched cottages at the fork, and look to the right, over the river, and you will see earthworks **(VII)** on the hillside – your last taste of history before welcome refreshment at the George, perhaps, or the Bourne Inn down the valley.

HISTORICAL and ARCHAEOLOGICAL NOTES
(multi-period)
Visits to the museums in Andover, Basingstoke, Newbury, Amesbury, Salisbury, and to Butser Ancient Farm are strongly recommended.
(I) St Mary Bourne: first documented in AD1185 as *(Capella de) Borne*, 'Stream' or 'On the River Borne'.

(II) Harrow Way branch track: prehistoric ridgeways ran E-W across S England, with smaller branch tracks linking them. The S-N branch track in this walk, running from Tidbury Ring to Walbury Hill (see map over), crossed the Harrow Way just west of Chapman's Ford, then headed northwards along the western ridge of the Bourne Valley.

(III) Portway Roman Road (AD43-409): Roman road running roughly NE-SW, from the important tribal centre at Silchester *(Calleva Atrebatum)* to Old Sarum *(Sorviodunum)*, and on to Dorchester *(Durnovaria)*. (See Walk 5).

(IV) Stone Age and Roman findspots: from the **Mesolithic** (BC10000-4001), three blade cores and ten tranchet axes (see *Glossary*) were found, now in Hampshire County Council Collections, Chilcomb House. A **Neolithic** (BC4000-2201) flint scraper and a fragment of polished stone axe are in storage in West Berkshire Museum, Newbury, though prehistoric artefacts from other sites are on display. **Roman** (AD43-409) pottery was found on the line of the Portway, in Derrydown Copse and when the lake was being dug, including New Forest ware, Oxfordshire ware, Alice Holt ware and Samian ware (see *Glossary* 'Roman Pottery').

(V) Rich findspot of Stone Age tools and implements in Breach Field on private land: from the **Palaeolithic** (BC500,000-10001), two handaxes and eight flint implements; from the **Mesolithic** (BC10000-4001), nine tranchet axes (see *Glossary*), three cores, two blades and flakes, and a pick, formerly in the collection of JB Stevens, now stored in Reading Museum; a scatter of **Neolithic** (BC4000-2201) flint implements; some **Bronze Age** (BC2200-801) scrapers and a distinctively-shaped barbed and tanged arrowhead. Andover Museum of the Iron Age, the Willis Museum, Basingstoke, and The Salibury Museum have impressive displays of Stone Age tools, including handaxes and tranchet axes, and Bronze Age barbed and tanged arrowheads, from other sites.

(VI) Findspot: Roman (AD43-409) pottery and building material discovered in a field by a local inhabitant.

(VII) Earthworks: undated terraces and lynchets (see *Glossary*), part of a field system, clearly visible on the hillside. Medieval or prehistoric.

Palaeolithic BC500,000-10001 Mesolithic 10000-4001	Neolithic BC4000-2201	Bronze Age BC2200-801	Iron Age BC800-AD42

Roman AD43-409	Early Med/Saxon AD410-1065	Medieval AD1066-1539	Post-Med AD1540-1900

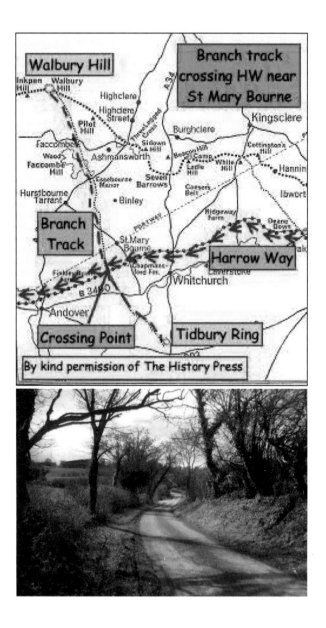

Walbury Hill

Branch track crossing HW near St Mary Bourne

Branch Track

Harrow Way

Crossing Point

Tidbury Ring

By kind permission of The History Press

27

Watery scenes in the Bourne Valley ...

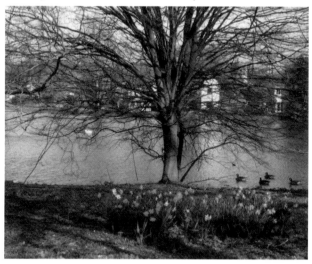

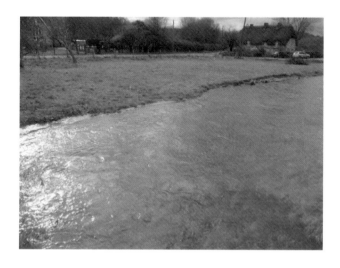

WALK 2: Setting the Scene

HARROW WAYFARERS in the NEOLITHIC (BC4000-2201)

Around BC3500, settlers arrived on our shores from the Continent, bringing with them the knowledge and practice of agriculture. These New Stone Age farmers cultivated wheat and barley, reared cattle, pigs and sheep, and made pots from clay - distinctive Grooved ware (see *Glossary* 'Neolithic Pottery'). They would have used the high ridges that radiate out from Salisbury Plain, to take stock to pasture on the unusually-open chalk down-land, and to trade with one another.

Items of breathtaking beauty would have changed hands along the Harrow Way - at that time probably just a local track. Polished stone axes, such as the greenstone axe found near Appleshaw, were exchanged over long distances, as trade was taking place not only locally but nationally and internationally. These prestige objects were not intended for everyday use, but perhaps as symbols of wealth and power, and to accompany the dead into the afterlife.

Our Neolithic Harrow Wayfarers were not only farmers and traders, but also monument builders, as this was the age of the long barrow. These communal burial mounds, such as Nutbane Long Barrow, made a statement in the landscape, and may have served as boundary markers as well as shrines for ancestor worship, often over many generations, before a ritual act of closure.

And perhaps our Harrow Wayfarers were heading for Salisbury Plain, where an early henge (see *Glossary*) consisting of a circular ditch with inner and outer banks, and a ring of blue stones from the Preseli Hills, was constructed around BC3000.

We can only guess at the arcane rituals that took place in these sacred spaces. If only our Neolithic Harrow Wayfarers could whisper their secrets ...

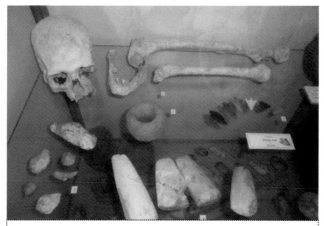

Skeletal remains and finds from Nutbane Long Barrow and surrounding area, courtesy of Andover Museum of the Iron Age, Hampshire Cultural Trust

WALK 2 ROUTE MAP (see OS Explorer 131)

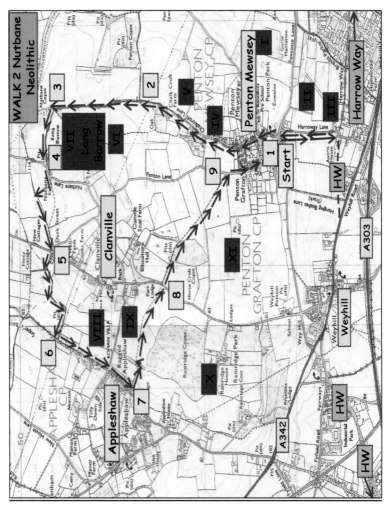

© Crown copyright and database rights 2021 OS Licence 100059949

WALK 2: NUTBANE, Penton Mewsey
Focus on the NEOLITHIC (BC4000-2201)

From Harrow Way to Neolithic long barrow

Over 6000 years of history lie around you on this walk. It brings you face to face with the Neolithic occupant of Nutbane Long Barrow (through a visit to Andover Museum) and passes close to the site (visible only on aerial photographs) of the communal funerary monument where he was laid to rest, over 5500 years ago. As this stretch of the Harrow Way lies either close to an industrial estate, or is lost entirely, the walk follows a S-N branch track that may once, perhaps, have linked the two contenders for the title 'Britain's Oldest Road' (see Note (IV) at end of walk).

Practical Information:

Distance: approx **8.5km/5.3miles+initial extension of 1km/0.6miles. Easy/Moderate.**

Parking: Roadside, by cricket ground in Chalkcroft Lane, Penton Mewsey.

Refreshments/Toilets: White Hart Inn, Penton Mewsey. Short drive to Fairground Café, Weyhill. No public toilets.

Terrain: Village and country lanes, bridleways, footpaths (may be muddy), tracks, short stretch on pavements. Dogs on lead, where indicated. Mainly level, apart from Harroway Lane extension.

Map: OS Explorer 131 Romsey, Andover & Test Valley.

Grid ref at start point: SU330 472

Best time of year: Bluebell time, for the azure carpet in Nutbane Copse.

32

About the Walk:

You step straight from the modern world into a quintessential English village, but you walk out into a much older landscape, where Bronze Age and Neolithic people buried their dead, and Romano-British elite built luxurious villas. So there are ancient footsteps to be followed, and scenes to be evoked, as you enjoy this pleasant ramble along footpaths, bridleways and country lanes, to meet the ancestors.

Highlights from the Neolithic:

>*site of long barrow (ploughed out)*
>*skeletal remains and finds in Andover Museum*
>*findspot of polished stone axe ('Thames Pick')*

Highlights from other periods:
>*site of extensive Bronze Age barrow cemetery*
>*sites of three Roman villas*
>*site of six Saxon or Medieval burials*

Imagine the Scene in the Neolithic:

One midsummer dawn over 5500 years ago, two prominent male members of the local community, and a child on the cusp of adulthood, were being laid to rest on the tribal boundary at Nutbane. They were being carefully placed, in a crouched position, on a bed of brushwood, in a timber mortuary structure, on the chalk-land north of the river. No feasting, just a simple ceremony of commemoration. Hundreds of years, and many more communal burials, later, there would be a ritual act of closure, and the dead would sleep, beneath a mound of soil and stones, for eternity.

START: The walk starts approx **1.5km** east of Weyhill, on the southern edge of **Penton Mewsey/Grafton (I).** Turn up **Chalkcroft Lane**, opposite Penton Village Hall, crossing the old brick bridge by the ford. Roadside parking should be possible by the cricket ground on the left. Please park sensitively.

Harroway Lane extension:

Before starting the main walk, if you wish to make the link with the **Harrow Way**, from the parking place return the short distance to the main road, cross **with great care**, and just round the bend, opposite the bus shelter, you will spot **Harroway Lane**, leading up to the ancient ridgeway. You may choose to walk up Harroway Lane for approx **500m** (not scenic and can be busy with traffic, especially at weekends), to the sharp bend, where the startling green shape of Harroway Cottage looms in front of you. Up here, the track joining from the left/east is the **Harrow Way,** a bridleway, and part of the Brenda Parker Way (see p35). The **Harrow Way** westward to Weyhill is lost, though the line of its continuation can be made out on the sharp bend near Harroway Cottage. To save yourself the uphill slog from the main road, however, you may prefer just to content yourself with a look at the photo of the **Harrow Way** on p46! But whether or not you choose to add this kilometre at the outset, you should pause to reflect on the vibrant archaeological landscape that lies alongside Harroway Lane (II) (III). Although there are no visible burial mounds to the south of the main road, if you take a few steps beyond the bus shelter on the main road, in the corner of Penton Park (private land) a **Bronze Age tumulus** should be clearly visible, topped with trees.

(1) From the foot of Harroway Lane on the main road, go back over the **old bridge by the ford** into the village. The spring that rises on the left marks the start of a tributary of the River Anton, which flows into the Test. Set off up **Chalkcroft Lane**, passing the entrance to 18[th]century Penton Lodge on the right, enjoying the quiet, picturesque village of **Penton Mewsey**. As you head northwards, you might like to imagine those Neolithic mourners, leaving the **Harrow Way** to follow an old south-north branch track **(IV)**, heading for Nutbane Long Barrow (see 'Imagine the Scene'). A visit to the 14[th]century Holy Trinity Church on the left is recommended, for the return journey, and, on a more secular note, to the White Hart Inn on the right. As the road bends round to the right, by the imposing **Old Rectory** on the left, follow a **No Through Road STRAIGHT AHEAD** (still Chalkcroft Lane).

Basically now just keep going straight, heading northwards up Chalkcroft Lane. The village lane becomes a **country lane/bridleway** beyond the small industrial estate of **Staddlestones Farm Units** on the left, and you will also notice the purple arrows of the **Brenda Parker Way**, a 78mile long-distance trail, in memory of a remarkable lady, whose invaluable contributions to country walking in this area can be viewed on the website. Beyond Chalk Croft Farm (V) the lane is less well-maintained, and may be muddy in places. Please keep dogs on lead, as indicated. A cool tunnel of native trees gives shade or shelter, eventually leading out onto farmland, with an open field on your left, and, shortly afterwards, a **barn** on your right.

(2)Pass to the left of the barn, keeping straight on northwards along the track. You are heading further back into history, and prehistory, with each step. The large field on your left is the probable site of a Roman villa (VI), one of three on this walk, and you are getting closer to your Neolithic goal.

(3) As the public right of way ends, a **line of trees** comes in diagonally from the left, and **Nutbane Copse** stretches ahead. Pause at the corner, just before leaving the track, and look to your left, into the field that lies in the angle between the diagonal line of trees and Nutbane Copse. A couple of hundred metres into the field, though visible only as cropmarks on aerial photographs, lies the site of our walk's focus, Nutbane Long Barrow (VII) – see artist's impression p45. It may not have been comparable in size to Wayland's Smithy or West Kennet Long Barrow, near the Great Ridgeway, but Nutbane is of equal antiquity. Although nothing remains on the ground, so the eye of the imagination will be required, there is an impressive range of finds from the site, including skeletal remains of one of the occupants, in Andover Museum of the Iron Age - well worth a visit, to bring the ancient site alive (so to speak!). Please see photo p30, and artist's impression p45. Having taken your time to evoke the scene, your walk now continues in a westerly direction. Leave the track which you have been following since the start of the walk, and turn **LEFT** to follow a blue-arrowed **bridleway** along the southern edge of Nutbane Copse, where **bluebells** carpet the woodland floor in season. When you emerge from the trees, keeping the narrow belt of woodland on your left, follow the footpath at the edge of the field (the narrow stretch shortly may be a little overgrown in summer), until you come to the **road**. Continue **straight ahead** past **Nutbane Cottage** on the left, for approx **100m**, until you come to a **sharp bend to the left.**

(4) If you wish to shorten the walk, you could follow the road back south to Penton Grafton, down first Nutbane Lane then Penton Lane. If, however, you wish to continue, **leave the road** as it bends sharply left and continue **STRAIGHT AHEAD** (westwards), following the direction of the yellow arrow, along a grassy track for approx **80m** until you reach **a simple step-through stile on the right,** just before the start of a (very) overgrown garden. **Turn RIGHT through the stile** (there may be another yellow arrow pointing in this direction, as it seems to be the farmer's preferred route for walkers) and follow a grassy path at the field edge, with the overgrown garden on your left. Continue along the field edge, with a hedge on your left, until you come to a **telegraph pole with a yellow 'Danger of Death' notice** in the corner of the field. Turn **LEFT** here to follow a **broad grassy track**, with a field on your right and a hedge interspersed with oak trees on your left. Continue along the left edge of another field, until the rooftops of **Clanville** (mentioned in Domesday Book, see *Glossary*) come into view ahead, on the valley floor. Descend to the road.

(5) By a private house named St Margaret's Chapel (note bell-cote on roof), cross the road with **GREAT CARE**, and take the **lane opposite**, with four semi-detached houses on the left. At the top of the slope, **DON'T** follow the lane round to the right, but take the **bridleway** to the **LEFT** (may be muddy) as it winds across farmland, between hedges. At the top of the next slope, take the **LEFT fork,** along a sheltered, tree-lined stretch for approx **200m**, until you emerge into the open. Straight ahead, Quarley Hillfort can be glimpsed in the distance (see Walk 4). Follow the track round to the right, by a line of pylons, and down the slope, keeping an eye and ear open for buzzards.

(6) At the foot of the slope, a **byway** comes in from the right. Turn **LEFT** to follow this – pleasantly shady on a warm summer's day. This is one of the old drove roads converging on Weyhill for the Fair (see *Harrow Wayfarers in the Medieval Period* p111). It leads you down into **Ragged Appleshaw** – the 'ragged' may be a corruption of 'roe gate', referring to the Royal Deer Forest of Chute. As you come to the road, pause for a moment: approx 200m along the road on your left, leading back towards Clanville, is the site of a second Roman villa (VIII) (nothing visible on the ground and on private land, so not worth a detour). Opposite it, a Neolithic stone axe (IX) was found. At the crossroads, cross with care and go **STRAIGHT AHEAD,** signed Appleshaw, along the **pavement** for approx **350m,** until you come to an **Appleshaw Parish Council notice-board** on your right, by a telegraph pole, opposite a patch of rough ground.

(7) Cross the road, and look carefully for a **narrow footpath with yellow arrow** immediately to the left of **South View House**, which leads between gardens and round a lone silver birch in the middle of the path. Follow this footpath, going gradually uphill, with houses and gardens on the left, and an open field on the right. Aim for a belt of trees on the crest of the ridge. Away to your right, a line of low hills forms the eastern fringe of Salisbury Plain. At the top of the slope, go into the beeches, turn **LEFT** along a clear path through the trees for approx **100m,** watching very carefully for a **yellow arrow on the RIGHT,** which you should follow. Leave the shelter of the trees here to follow a **strip path through the crops**, with Ramridge

Copse on your right, and, beyond that, though not visible, Ramridge Park and House (X). Continue down through the field to the road.

(8) Cross the road with **GREAT CARE** and go through the **white picket gate** opposite, to the left of the large white gate, to take the **footpath**, sandwiched between a fence on the right and hedge on the left, with horses in the fields on both sides, (Clanville Stud Farm lies to the left). Where there are gaps in the hedge on the left, look for glimpses of the rather grand Blissamore Hall, formerly Clanville Lodge (visit website for more information). Continue into Horse Croft Copse ahead, with neatly-coppiced hazels arching over the path, shortly coming to a **white metal gate** on the left. Just beyond it, **go round the stile** and out into the open. A couple of fields away on the right, yet another Roman villa (XI) was discovered. Follow the footpath **STRAIGHT AHEAD** across two fields, back to the road.

(9) At the road, turn **RIGHT** to head down into the peaceful hamlet of **Penton Grafton,** for a final taste of the Neolithic. At an unspecified location, worked flints, including a 'Thames Pick' (see *Glossary*) were found, now on display in the Andover Museum of the Iron Age. At the foot of the slope, as the road bends to the left, the field beyond **Pear Tree Cottage** on the right is the possible site of a Shrunken Medieval Village (see *Glossary*). Passing the peaceful pool on your right, return to your vehicle by the cricket ground. Before heading for some refreshment at The White Hart Inn, you may like to visit Holy Trinity Church, tucked away beside the manor house. This 14[th]century building replaces an earlier one mentioned in Domesday.

HISTORICAL and ARCHAEOLOGICAL NOTES (multi-period)

A visit to Andover Museum of the Iron Age is essential, to view some of the finds relating to this walk, and to The Salisbury Museum.

(I) Penton Mewsey/Grafton: thought to derive from *Penitone,* meaning 'farm held at a penny rent', this village and hamlet are believed to date from the 10th/early 11[th]century, when Saxon landholders were attracted to the banks of the stream, and when other villages in the area, including Andover itself, began to appear out of what had been Royal Hunting Forest.

(II) Bronze Age barrow cemetery, east of Harroway Lane (BC2200-801): 14 or more ring ditches are clearly visible as cropmarks on aerial photographs. Their position, on rising ground overlooking the stream, is similar to other Bronze Age barrow cemeteries. Perhaps these sites were seen as an important part of the sacred landscape, with water sources forming a point of contact with the spirit world. Streams flowing east from their source, as here, may have been particularly special. On a more recent note, the Bronze Age barrow cemetery lies on the site of RAF Andover, a

41

former Royal Flying Corps and RAF station, from where OGS Crawford, first Archaeology Officer for Ordnance Survey, flew in the 1920s.

(III) Saxon or Medieval burials (AD410-1539): six graves were observed during excavations at Harroway Farm. Though their date is uncertain, a knife found with one of the burials is thought to be Saxon or Medieval.

(IV) Harrow Way branch track: prehistoric ridgeways ran E-W across S England, with smaller branch tracks linking them, as in Walk 1. Though undocumented, could there have been a S-N route here linking the Harrow Way with the N Hampshire Ridgeway, then west to join the Great Ridgeway? (See map *Wessex Ridgeways* in frontispieces). And could this, at least partially, explain the location of Nutbane Long Barrow?

(V) Roman pottery: Late Roman pottery (3rd-4thcentury), including New Forest ware (see *Glossary*) and grey tempered ware, were recovered near Chalk Croft Farm.

(VI) Roman villa site (AD43-409): Roman brick, debris, a short stretch of flint walling, along with Roman pottery (coarse black gritted ware and some Samian sherds) indicated the site nearby of a possible Roman villa. The rich farmland of this area was ideal for cereals production, in Roman times as today. Five villa sites to the west of Andover were identified in the 1880s-90s, including this one, to the east of Clanville, and at Appleshaw (see **Note VIII**).

42

(VII) Site of Nutbane Neolithic Long Barrow (BC4000-2201): partially excavated in 1957 by the superbly-named Faith de Mallet Morgan, for the Andover History Group, this heavily-ploughed burial mound, approx 52m in length, revealed the former existence of a **forecourt enclosure**, and two free-standing **mortuary structures**, each with more than one construction phase. A date of **BC3500** was given for one of the **later** construction phases. **Four crouched burials were found in the timber structure at the east end, placed on a layer of light brushwood: a male, 5'9", aged 30-40; a second male, 5'6", aged 40-50, and a child aged 12-13.** At a later date, a **fourth male was added, aged 30-40.** Eventually there would have been a **ceremonial act of closure**, burying the mortuary structures beneath a mound of soil and stones from flanking ditches. The long barrow may have served as a tribal boundary marker, and a focus for ancestor worship.

(VIII) Roman villa site: late 3rd-4th century Romano-British villa, where a large courtyard and three detached wings were excavated by the Rev. GH Engleheart in 1897. Mosaic floors, *Opus Signinum* (see *Glossary*) pavements, and hypocaust heating systems were found, indicating a degree of affluence and comfort.

(IX) Neolithic axe findspot (BC4000-2201): a polished greenstone axe, with a diagonal band of quartz around the butt end, is stored in The Salisbury Museum, where a rare and beautiful

Early Neolithic jadeite axe from near Stonehenge is usually on display.

(X) Ramridge House and Park: originally a religious house, granted by William the Conqueror to the Abbey of Grestayn in Normandy. At the end of the 14[th]century, Geoffrey Chaucer owned Ramridge Manor and the site of the Weyhill Fair. The present (private) house dates from c1740.

(XI) Roman villa site (AD43-409): a scatter of Roman building materials, including roof slabs, flue tiles and floor tiles, was found in a field, along with a quern, pottery and burnt flint.

Palaeolithic BC500,000-10001 Mesolithic 10000-4001	Neolithic BC4000-2201	Bronze Age BC2200-801	Iron Age BC800-AD42

Roman AD43-409	Early Med/Saxon AD410-1065	Medieval AD1066-1539	Post-Med AD1540-1900

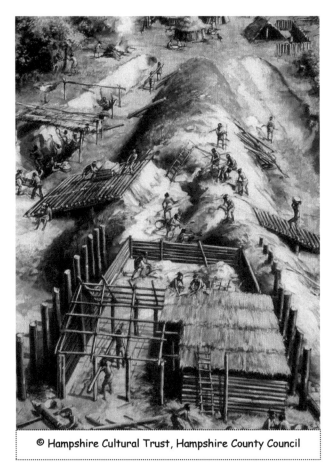

Artist's impression of the construction of Nutbane Long Barrow. From a painting by Mike Codd, courtesy of Hampshire Cultural Trust

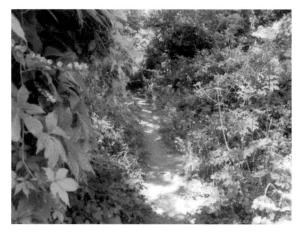

*Harrow Way at the top of Harroway Lane,
looking east*

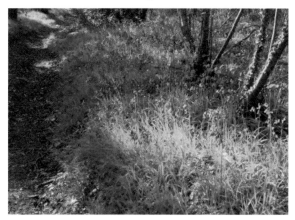

Nutbane Copse bluebells between **(3)** *and* **(4)**

WALK 3: Setting the Scene

HARROW WAYFARERS in the BRONZE AGE (BC2200-801)

The Golden Age of the Harrow Way - literally!

Around BC2500 a wave of migrants, termed the Beaker people (see *Glossary*), had arrived on our shores from Central Europe, bringing with them metalworking skills. Copper, initially, was to topple the supremacy of stone, for tools, weapons and prestige items, until, around BC2200, it was discovered that copper mixed with tin gave a stronger metal alloy – bronze. Good news for Britain, as we shall see.

By the Bronze Age, the prehistoric local ridgeways were starting to link up into a network of routes, to cater for national and international trade. Britain's mineral wealth was of great importance. In addition to tin in Cornwall, copper came from Great Orme Head in North Wales, lead from the Mendips, gold from Wales and Ireland. The Harrow Way was of strategic importance for conveying these ores and minerals across Southern England. By the Bronze Age, trade was 'big business', and those who controlled the flow of copper and tin became rich.

As well as raw materials, prestige items were changing hands along the Harrow Way, some of which accompanied the dead to their burials in the distinctive round barrows that dotted the horizon. These usually contained one important individual, though sometimes more, often accompanied by items of breathtaking beauty, such as the two pairs of delicate gold earrings accompanying two men into the afterlife, in a burial at Chilbolton, south of the Harrow Way (see Andover Museum of the Iron Age).

Bronze hoards have been found in the Andover area, one of which was discovered, in the early 19th century, in watercress beds in the River Anton. A careless moment or an act of devotion, venerating the gods?

Ritual must have been such an integral part of Bronze Age lives that they were prepared to travel great distances to attend ceremonies – isotopic analysis shows that at Durrington Walls, near Stonehenge, the pigs being feasted upon came from the Scottish Highlands. Did our Harrow Wayfarers include weary pigs? Quite possibly.

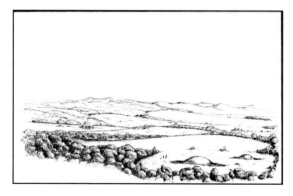

Line drawing of Bronze Age landscape,
with thanks to David Hopkins

48

WALK 3 ROUTE MAP (see OS Explorer 144)

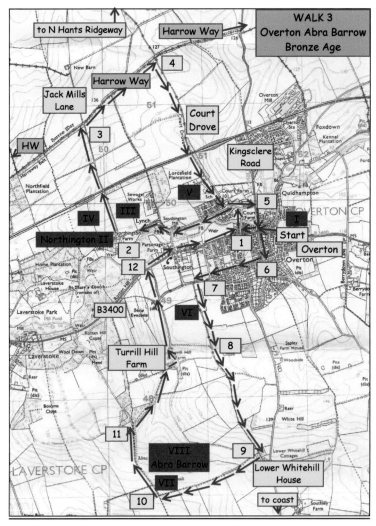

© Crown copyright and database rights 2021 OS Licence 100059949

WALK 3: OVERTON Abra Barrow
Focus on the BRONZE AGE (BC2200-801)

From Harrow Way to Bronze Age barrows

Overton (see Walk 8 Note (I)) is an attractive village on the Test with a flourishing present and evidence of occupation going back thousands of years. As a particularly fine stretch of Harrow Way runs across the parish two kilometres to the north, Overton is used as the base for two walks. The village lies close to a meeting of ancient tracks, with the E-W line of the Harrow Way crossed by a S-N route, heading up over the downs to join the North Hampshire Ridgeway.

Practical Information:

Distance:approx **14km/8.7miles. Challenging.**

Parking: Free car park in London Street, at the recycling centre by Turnpike Cottages, about 200m east of the crossroads and traffic lights in the centre of the village.

Refreshments/Toilets: Good choice of tea rooms and pubs in Overton. No public toilets.

Terrain: Easy walking on chalk-and-flint tracks, quiet country roads, woodland footpaths and green lanes (may be muddy). Some ascents and descents.

Map:OS Explorer 144 Basingstoke, Alton & Whitchurch.

Grid ref at start point:SU517 497

Best time of year: Enjoyable at any time of year, though some stretches exposed in winter. Harrow Way quieter Nov-May (no off-road vehicles).

About the Walk

An exhilarating figure-of-eight walk across rolling down-land with far-reaching views, extending from the Harrow Way on the northern horizon to the barrow-topped ridge to the south. From the centre of Overton it follows the Test westwards, climbs to join the Harrow Way - a delightful green lane - before returning to the village down an old drove road. It then heads south along an ancient trackway up onto the downs, to reach an extensive Bronze Age barrow cemetery, where Abra Barrow rises majestically right beside the road. With thanks to the landowner of Laverstoke Park Farm.

Highlights from the Bronze Age:

>Abra Barrow, a large, visible, burial mound
>extensive Bronze Age ritual site, in a prehistoric landscape
>ancient trackway from the Harrow Way to a barrow cemetery

Highlights from other periods:
>Neolithic flint axe findspot
>findspot of three Roman pottery vessels, black-burnished ware (see Glossary 'Roman Pottery')
>site of Iron Age, Roman and Saxon settlements

Imagine the Scene in the Bronze Age:

Follow in the footsteps of a group of Bronze Age mourners, heading south from the Harrow Way, down to cross the river, then up to the downs beyond, to attend a ceremony in commemoration of a well-loved chieftain, in the barrow cemetery on the crest of the ridge.

51

Before leaving the car park in London Street, by Turnpike Cottages, look over to the playground and the housing development to the right, where an **important archaeological site (I)** was discovered, now buried beneath the residential area.

START: Make your way downhill to the **crossroads by the** White Hart Inn (see Walk 8 Note (X)), cross at the **lights** to the coffee shop on the corner opposite, and walk **STRAIGHT AHEAD** (west) along **High Street**. Over to the right a **Roman cremation** was found, and **three Roman pottery vessels** were amongst the first items deposited with Winchester Museum in 1853, now stored in Hampshire County Council Collections at Chilcomb House (see p164). Continue past Overton Gallery on the right (well worth a visit and tea stop later) until you come to **Bridge Street** on the right.

(1) Turn **RIGHT** up **Bridge Street**, passing pretty cottages, some with riverside gardens, over the little bridge, where it may have been possible to ford the young Test in prehistoric times. Continue past the Sports Ground on the right, until you come to the **Old Rectory** on the corner – a mid-19th century Gothic mansion. Ahead is the warm brick serenity of Court Farmhouse (see Walk 8 Note (IX)) where the Medieval manorial court was held. Turn **LEFT** at the **Old Rectory** into **Court Drove,** go past Glebe Gardens on the left, and on up the hill. **Leave Court Drove** at the corner where it makes a sharp right turn, and continue **STRAIGHT AHEAD** along **Silk Mill Lane,** where the first water-powered silk mill in Southern England was built in 1769 (now demolished). This quiet lane runs along the north bank of the Test, with glimpses through the trees of lawns and sunlight glinting on water. Continue past **Southington Lane**, which joins from the left, and go **STRAIGHT AHEAD** along the **No Through Road** (The Lynch) which will take you, in time, past Southington Mill on the left, a former 18[th]century corn mill, now a private house, and beyond the house, the Post-Medieval mill race and sluices. Follow the lane round until it eventually comes to an end at Northington Farm, all that remains of the Deserted Medieval Village (see *Glossary*) of Northington (II).

(2) At Northington Farm, where the road ends, turn **RIGHT** up the track that gradually climbs, between hedges. Over in the fields on the right, prehistoric activity **(III)** was uncovered during an archaeological evaluation of the area near the Water Treatment Works. In the field on your left lies a probable Romano-British site **(IV)**. Carry on over the **railway bridge** until you eventually reach a **crossing of tracks.** Go **STRAIGHT AHEAD** to follow **a footpath, signed with a red byway arrow,** as it climbs between sheltering hedges, heading for the **Harrow Way** on the ridge. After approx **400m** you come to another **crossing of**

tracks **by a wooden signpost**, indicating **byway** to left and right, and **Jack Mills Lane** straight on. You have reached the Harrow Way.

(3)Turn RIGHT here to follow this ancient trackway north-eastwards through a belt of deciduous woodland, bounded by banks separating it from the surrounding farmland. These banks are indicators of the old drove road (see *Glossary*). A brooding silence hangs in the air, between centuries-old oaks and beeches, draped in pendulous creepers. Ignore any footpaths joining the Harrow Way until you eventually reach – approx **1km** from the Jack Mills Lane crossroads – a **footpath crossing the** Harrow Way, **and a wooden signpost with a red arrow tacked on halfway down. Concrete barriers may be in position, and there are two No Entry road signs for cars Nov-May.** This is the point at which you leave the Harrow Way.

(4) Turn **RIGHT** here to leave the Harrow Way and head back towards Overton down **Court Drove**, shown on the OS map. You might like to imagine the Bronze Age footsteps which you will be following all the way to the **barrow cemetery** on the southern horizon (see 'Imagine the Scene'). Court Drove makes for a pleasant, sheltered walk across open farmland, with the ploughed-out site of a Bronze Age ring ditch, possibly surrounding a tumulus, over in the fields to the right. There is a gentle descent to cross the **railway bridge**, entering Overton by the Primary School, in the grounds of which a Mesolithic findspot (V) is located. Continue down the road, retracing the steps of your outward journey until you reach the Old Rectory on the right. Don't turn down Bridge Street this time, but continue **STRAIGHT AHEAD,** passing the Church of St Mary (visit website) on your left, to the **T-junction**.

(5) At the T-junction turn **RIGHT** to take you back down Kingsclere Road to the traffic lights at the **crossroads by the White Hart** in the centre of the village – time for some refreshment before starting the southern loop of the walk.
From the traffic lights head **STRAIGHT ACROSS** (south) for approx **250m** up **Winchester Street**, admiring the old cottages on either side, dating from the 15th-19thcenturies.

(6) When you reach the **Greyhound Inn** on the right, a Neolithic flint axe was found close by, now stored in the Willis Museum, Basingstoke. Turn **RIGHT** into **Greyhound Lane,** up the short, steep slope, then continue **STRAIGHT AHEAD** along **Dellands,** through a quiet residential area for approx **600m**, until the road makes a sharp bend to the right, by a short terrace of attractive cottages on the left. Leave the road at the corner to go **STRAIGHT AHEAD along a track,** an old, sunken byway between high, tree-topped banks – an indication of its antiquity. In spring and summer, look out for dormice nesting boxes hanging in the trees – please, of course, leave undisturbed. After approx **150m** you come to a small triangle of grass and a **T-junction**, where a footpath joins from the right.

(7) Turn **LEFT at the T-junction** to head south along a **byway** which is an ancient trackway (VI). On the left, as you go up the gradual slope, lies the site of Medieval/Post-Medieval brickworks, where a 13th-14thcentury lead seal was found. Basically, now, just keep going straight, following what is sometimes a track, sometimes a narrower footpath, enjoying the shelter of the old banks and hedges, white with blossom in season, with sloes and blackberries later.

(8) You eventually emerge from this sheltered, tree-lined footpath by a **barn** on the right, passing a chalk track that joins from the right. **Keeping to the left of the barn,** take the unsurfaced track **STRAIGHT AHEAD,** which shortly becomes tree-lined again. When you come out of the trees, you will see that the track **bends round to the left**, and ahead stretches a **large hedge** (at the time of writing). Leave the track at the corner where the hedge starts, by a metal gate into a field on the left, and continue **STRAIGHT AHEAD**, keeping the **hedge on your left**, following a grassy bridleway up a gradual incline. This is exposed down-land, and the hedge provides welcome shelter from east winds. Carry on over the crest of the ridge, and down to where a **cluster of beeches** screens **Lower**

Whitehill House, (marked as Cottages on the OS Map) approx **1km** south of the barn you passed earlier. The trees are on your left, in the garden, where you may also spot a **tree house**, though the name of Lower Whitehill House is not visible.

(9) At the entrance to Lower Whitehill House, (an attractive red brick building), there is a **five bar gate across the track.** Turn **RIGHT** immediately before the gate, to join a **farm road** that will take you westwards across high, lonely farmland. The land belongs to Laverstoke Park Farm (visit website – most interesting – and you might even spot a distant buffalo!). For the next kilometre – the entire stretch from **(9) to (10)** – the fields on the right are the site of an extensive Bronze Age barrow cemetery. As the hedge ends, look to your right, and your first burial mound is just visible, at the top of the field. Although the majority of the burial mounds have been ploughed out, not quite all.

(10) After approx **1km,** the road makes a **sharp bend to the right**. Look carefully in the corner of the field on the right, and a round barrow (VII) is just visible as a low ridge, approx 100m from the southern hedge, and slightly closer to the western, therefore best viewed once you have rounded the corner and are heading up the road towards the crest. This whole area, between the road you are currently on, and the track you came up, was a sacred place 4000 years ago - a focus for burials and ceremonies commemorating ancestors and tribal leaders – and reachable from the Harrow Way, the line of which can just be seen on the northern horizon. Continue up the lane, looking ahead for your first glimpse of ABRA BARROW (VIII), which is right beside the road, in the top corner of the field. Though on private land, it is so close that you have a good view. The sites of a further nine barrows (ploughed out) are close by – clearly a prominent position near the crest of the ridge was important to the Bronze Age barrow builders. And this area may already have had ritual significance long before the Bronze Age, as a Neolithic flint axe and three scrapers were found near the site of Abra Barrow.

(11)Having evoked the Bronze Age scene in the mind's eye, continue north-eastwards towards Overton, following the farm road down into the valley to Turrill Hill Farm. Pause, perhaps, by the farm to look back up at the ridge. Although Abra Barrow itself is no longer visible, it is just possible to make out the adjacent gap in the hedge, where the road disappears over the crest. Carry on up the road to the right of the house, and now just keep going. Approx 800m after Turrill Hill Farm, the country road descends to join the main road, B3400, named Rotten Hill here.

(12)Cross the main road WITH GREAT CARE, to the pavement on the far side, turning RIGHT to head back into the centre of Overton (just over 1km), for some refreshment.

HISTORICAL and ARCHAEOLOGICAL NOTES (multi-period)

Visits to the museums in Andover and Basingstoke are strongly recommended.

(I) Iron Age, Roman and Saxon settlements (BC800-AD1065), including a sunken-featured Saxon building (see *Glossary*), where evidence suggesting a small textile industry was found, including a spindle whorl, loom-weight fragments and a bone pin.

(II) Northington: Deserted Medieval Village (see *Glossary*) first documented in AD1218. Northington had been a substantial village with 35 households or more, which, by 1485, had shrunk to four tenants. In that year the Bishop of Winchester leased the land to William Ayliffe, who was to build a new house on the site of the cottage of one of the last four tenants. He was also to enclose the arable land of the village into four fields.

(III) Prehistoric pits: one contained dog's teeth and some probable Beaker (see *Glossary*) pottery from the Late Neolithic/Early Bronze Age (BC2500-2200). Earlier Mesolithic and Neolithic struck flints were also found.

(IV) Romano-British temple and buildings (AD43-409): a square enclosure interpreted as a Romano-British temple, along with the foundations of several other buildings, visible as cropmarks on aerial photographs.

(V) Mesolithic tranchet axe (BC10000-4001) (see *Glossary*): in storage in The Salisbury Museum.

Good examples from other sites are on display in the museums in Andover and Basingstoke.

(VI) Ancient trackway: prehistoric branch track, running S-N, crossing the E-W line of the Harrow Way, linking the North Hants Ridgeway with the South Coast.

(VII) Bronze Age round barrow, surviving as a low ridge (BC2200-801): the barrow cemetery extended from Abra Barrow right across to where Lower Whitehill House now stands.

(VIII) ABRA BARROW (BC2400-1500): large Bronze Age bowl barrow (see *Glossary*), c32m in diameter, on the crest of a low chalk ridge. Roughly circular, with a central mound about 1.8m high, it is enclosed to the SE by an in-filled ditch. Its commanding position suggests it was intended to be seen from a distance. A ring ditch is visible as a cropmark on aerial photographs. No grave goods were revealed.

Palaeolithic BC500,000-10001 Mesolithic 10000-4001	Neolithic BC4000-2201	Bronze Age BC2200-801	Iron Age BC800-AD42

Roman AD43-409	Early Med/Saxon AD410-1065	Medieval AD1066-1539	Post-Med AD1540-1900

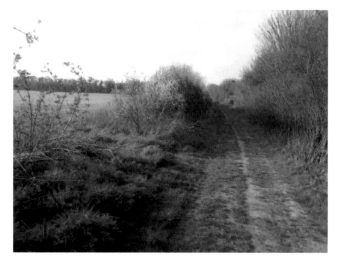

*Court Drove near **(4)** with the Harrow Way
marked by a line of trees on the skyline*

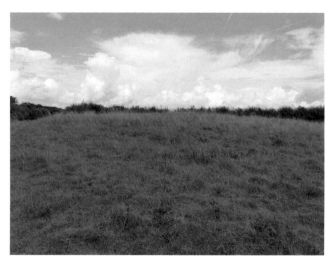

*Abra Barrow, between **(10)** and **(11)***

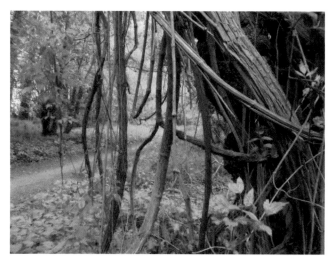

Pendulous creepers by the Harrow Way near (3)

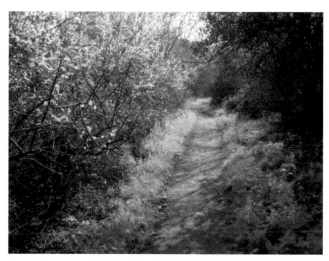

Ancient trackway near (7) leading south to the Bronze Age barrow cemetery

WALK 4: Setting the Scene
HARROW WAYFARERS in the IRON AGE (BC800-AD42)

In the Iron Age, as in previous millennia, Harrow Wayfarers would have included farmers, trundling along in ox-drawn carts to reach their terraced fields. These were larger now than the patchwork of small fields in the Bronze Age, thanks to the increased efficiency and robustness of iron-tipped ploughs, incorporating the new metalworking technologies that had arrived from the East.

Our Iron Age Harrow Wayfarers would have lived in thatched timber roundhouses, in larger settlements than in the Bronze Age, surrounded by palisaded enclosures where cattle and sheep were reared, along with pigs, small horses and domestic fowl. Barley, oats, wheat and the new seed beans were cultivated, in 'Celtic' field systems (see *Glossary*). Some communities had banjo enclosures (see *Glossary*) - funnel-shaped constructions probably used to hold or herd livestock.

Along the Harrow Way, farmers might have been making their way to **Quarley Hillfort,** perhaps to attend a ceremonial gathering, or to trade brightly-coloured woollen cloth for seeds of the new spelt wheat that was replacing emmer. The first hillforts had begun to appear in the Late Bronze Age, from around BC1000, when a deterioration in climate, combined with an increase in population, put pressure on the landscape, probably making it necessary to define and display ownership of land.

Hillforts were of strategic importance in the landscape, and formed part of a network. Quarley Hill stands at a meeting of ancient ways. Crossing the east-west line of the Harrow Way, a north-south route led southwards to Danebury (guarding the crossing of the River Test) and northwards to Sidbury Hill, before branching west to join the Great Ridgeway and east along the North Hampshire Ridgeway to the North Downs.

This NW Hampshire down-land was clearly a busy place at the time, and its story is admirably told in Andover Museum of the Iron Age.

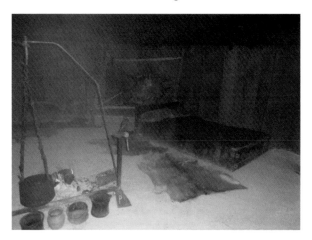

Inside a reconstructed Iron Age roundhouse,
courtesy of Butser Ancient Farm

WALK 4 ROUTE MAP (see OS Explorer 131)

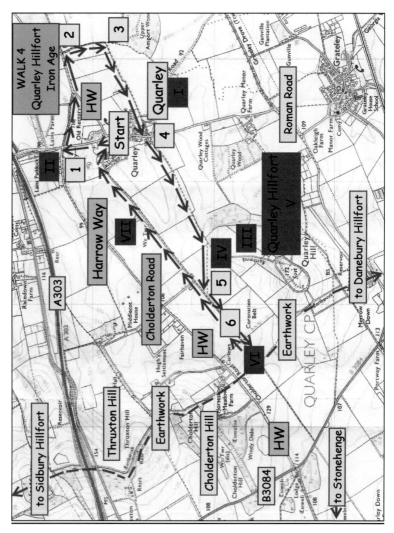

© Crown copyright and database rights 2021 OS Licence 100059949

WALK 4: QUARLEY HILL
Focus on the IRON AGE (BC800-AD42)

From Harrow Way to hillfort, through an Iron Age agricultural landscape

Seen from the east, **Quarley Hill** rises like a beacon – part of a line of hills forming the eastern approaches to Salisbury Plain. Some, like Quarley, and Sidbury to the north, would acquire hillforts in the Iron Age. For the ancient travellers along the Harrow Way, this would have been an awe-inspiring landscape, heralding the great ceremonial centres of the Plain. Long before Iron Age farmers managed the chalk down-land, Mesolithic and Neolithic people made use of the natural resources. Bronze Age earthworks converge here, and, later, a major Roman road passed close by.

Practical Information:

Distance:approx **7km/4.3miles. Easy.**

Parking: Quarley Village Hall, if not in use, or roadside in the village.

Public transport: Stagecoach bus number 5 stops in the village. Visit website.

Refreshments/Toilets: Cholderton Farm Shop & Café, and Crown Inn, Cholderton, close by. No public toilets.

Terrain: Level tracks, footpaths, country lanes. Two stiles. Dogs on lead where indicated.

Map:OS Explorer 131 Romsey, Andover & Test Valley.

Grid ref at start point:SU274 438

Best time of year:A day of breezy sunshine or moody skies, perhaps.

About the Walk:

An exhilarating, low-level, figure-of-eight walk, allowing the hillfort to be viewed from different angles. Approached from the east, it appears first as a tree-topped cone, rising above the fields; then, at closer quarters, a gentle giant, stretching along the contours, behind its single bank and ditch. There is only a moderate stretch of Harrow Way in this walk, to keep it off-road, but you follow footpaths and tracks through an ancient agricultural landscape associated with the prehistoric trackway, and as productive 2500 years ago as today. There is no public access to the summit of the hillfort, but views are magnificent. An old drove road completes the circuit, bringing you back into the village down one of its prettiest lanes.

Highlights from the Iron Age:

>hillfort, landmark for early travellers

>field systems and earthworks, visible as linear ditches in certain light and crop conditions

>sites of two Iron Age settlements and banjo enclosures (see Glossary)

Highlights from other periods:

> Norman church with Saxon origins

>findspots of prehistoric tools and Roman pottery

>probable site of manor house, shown by earthworks

Imagine the Scene in the Iron Age:

Follow in the footsteps of an Iron Age farmer, leaving his thatched roundhouse in the large settlement beside the Harrow Way. He is

heading for the terraced fields at the foot of Quarley Hill, to till the land with the ox-drawn, iron-tipped ard (see *Glossary*) that he shares with his neighbours. He will plant the seed beans recently acquired at a springtime gathering up on the hillfort, in exchange for woollen cloth woven by his wife.

START: The walk starts in Quarley (I). The initial eastward loop from Quarley village enhances the experience of a distant landmark growing closer, and takes you along the Harrow Way. Before leaving the village hall car park, note the 'lumps and bumps' in the field between the hall and the church, and to the rear of the hall – in all likelihood the site of the manor house and associated buildings, where, it is claimed, the Prince Regent stayed. **From the parking place, head north** along the road to the Church of St Michael, 11th century but with Saxon origins (note the blocked-up doorway and windows in the nave). Approx **400m** from the village hall you come to a **junction** just before Lains Farm (II) by a quirky signpost, indicating the road to Cholderton to the left.

(1) Turn **RIGHT** here to leave the road and follow the tree-lined **footpath** (may be muddy). This is the Harrow Way. When the footpath emerges onto a quiet country lane (still the Harrow Way), continue **STRAIGHT AHEAD** until the road bends to the left.

68

(2) At the bend, **leave** the Harrow Way and turn **RIGHT** along a delightful, sheltered little **footpath**, winding its way between thickets of hawthorn, elder and ivy, with small clumps of violets in season. Follow in the footsteps of the Iron Age farmer, heading to the terraced fields at the foot of Quarley Hill (see 'Imagine the Scene').

(3) As the footpath emerges into a field, turn immediately **RIGHT** and follow the field edge back towards Quarley, keeping the tall hedge on your right. Enjoy views ahead of **Quarley Hill** – pleasingly rounded and, from this angle, symmetrical even down to the clumps of trees on its summit. Sense the anticipation of those early Harrow Wayfarers, knowing that this hillfort signified the gateway to the Stonehenge landscape, just over the horizon. Leave the field to head along by a terrace of quaintly-named thatched cottages, until you reach the road.

(4) Cross the road **WITH GREAT CARE** to a track leading to a barn. Immediately on the **left** is a **gate** into a field, with a **stile adjacent**. Cross the stile into the field. Dogs on lead, if indicated. Continue along the **right edge** of the field, heading for Quarley Hill. Cross another **stile,** bear **LEFT** into the corner of the **second** field, then round to the **RIGHT**, following the left edge of the field, with an old hedge on your left, dense with ivy, wild roses and fruit trees. Quarley Hill is hidden now, but there are good views ahead of tree-topped Cholderton Hill and, to its right, Thruxton Hill, though neither is crowned with a hillfort. On entering a **third** field, keep to the edge, with the hedge on your left, until you come to the end of the field, then pass through a **gap in the hedge ahead** into the top corner of the **fourth** field. Pause here, with the flanks of Quarley Hill rising on your left, and consider the thoughts of R. Hippisley Cox (see *References and Sources* p156) that the beacon-like appearance of the hill, when viewed from afar, is difficult to imagine when one is standing at the foot of its gentle slopes. Up to the left, evidence of the Romans was found **(III)** (Portway Roman Road runs just to the south of Quarley Hill). As you follow the **strip path diagonally across the field**, the hillfort on the summit gradually comes into view, and you cross an **earthwork**, visible in the correct light and crop conditions, heading north **(IV)**. Indeed the whole area is criss-crossed with prehistoric field and ranch boundaries, dating from the Bronze Age, and still very much in use by our Iron Age farmers.

(5) At the bottom of the field you come to a **broad grassy track**, and a simple but welcome **bench** (may be overgrown) allowing a brief rest, and time to take in the full magnificence of **Quarley Hillfort (V)** and the archaeology that surrounds it. Before turning back towards the village, you may like to head along the grassy track for approx **400m**, towards **Coronation Belt** (marked on the OS map), to gain the best view of the hillfort, where it is just possible to make out the **gap in the bank surrounding the summit of the hillfort**, below the trees. This gap faces the **Harrow Way**, which lies parallel to the track you are on. A short distance beyond Coronation Belt, look to your right, where a bungalow can be seen beside the **Harrow Way**/Cholderton Road at the foot of Cholderton Hill. Another **linear ditch/earthwork** crosses the track you are on, again visible only in the right conditions (depending on the time of year, angle of the sun and crop growth), thought to mark a **crossing of ancient ways (VI)**. Marked on the OS map, it runs to the left of where the bungalow now stands, up and over Cholderton Hill, skirting the woods on its summit. Before turning for home, the rambler might be drawn on up the grassy track to the crest of the ridge, from where views open out to the west, towards Salisbury Plain. On a breezy day, this is exhilarating, open down-land.

(6) Retrace your steps to the little bench, then **STRAIGHT ON** along the grassy track, heading back towards Quarley village. This track has all the features of a **Medieval drove road**, broad and green, with low banks or tall hedges of old yews separating it from the surrounding farmland, to funnel stock in one direction. In this case, that direction would have been to the Weyhill Fair (see *Harrow Wayfarers in the Medieval Period* p111). The drove road runs parallel to the **Harrow Way**, a field's width away to the left, now the minor road

71

from Quarley to Cholderton. In the distance, beyond the Harrow Way, traffic on the A303 thunders westwards. On the left you pass the site of further Iron Age field boundaries, then, in the belt of trees on the left, another Iron Age site (VII). This was clearly a busy and well-populated area in the Iron Age. Continue back along the track, as it becomes a metalled lane, leading down into the village past picturesque early 18thcentury cottages, thatched and timber-framed. Pass the war memorial and bus stop, then round the corner to the village hall.

HISTORICAL and ARCHAEOLOGICAL NOTES (multi-period)

Visits to Andover Museum of the Iron Age and Butser Ancient Farm are highly recommended.

(I) Quarley village: some sources maintain that *Ferlei* ('Clearing in a Wood') was first mentioned in Domesday Book (1086), whilst others believe that the first documentary evidence of *Cornelea* ('Clearing or Wood with Querns or Mills') is in 1167. It is possible that the Saxon King Athelstan, grandson of Alfred, billeted his troops here, during the celebrations accompanying his victory tour of England in AD928, after announcing his Code of Laws in nearby Grateley.

(II) Large-scale Iron Age settlement beneath Lains Farm (BC800-AD42): three enclosures, including a possible banjo enclosure (see *Glossary*). 16 pits were excavated, probably used for storage. Two pits contained loom-weights and a large amount of **pottery**. A structure built on top of one of the pits is probably an **oven**, used for parching grain. To the north of Lains Farm, by the A303, lies the site of an Iron Age quarry where a **Roman inhumation** was found. The grave of a supine young male was cut into the quarry scoop, with no trace of a coffin, but accompanied by two items of New Forest ware (see *Glossary* 'Roman Pottery'). Probably part of a cemetery.

(III) Roman pottery (AD43-409) found in considerable quantities.

(IV) Late Bronze Age linear ditch (BC1200-801): excavation in 1938 established that these banks and ditches were earlier than the Iron Age hillfort, as its ramparts were built over and through them. They may have been associated with control, ownership and use of the land.

(V) Quarley Iron Age Hillfort: a univallate (single ditch) hillfort, dated by pottery to BC5th-3rdcenturies. There is limited evidence of occupation, so this may have been short-lived. It is likely that the two settlements near the Harrow Way were where the community lived, with the hillfort being used primarily as a meeting place. Quarley was part of a network of hillforts, with Danebury to the SE and Sidbury to the NW. Portway Roman Road (see Walk 5) runs along the southern edge of the hill. Prehistoric findspots surround the hillfort. On the southern bank of the hillfort, a Mesolithic flint core, which would have produced very fine blades, was found, now in Exeter Museum, and on

the NE edge, a **leaf-shaped Neolithic blade.**
Bronze Age flint tools, including **two scrapers, a blade and a fragment of polished axe**, were found to the SE of the hillfort. To the SW lies a **Late Bronze Age linear ditch and ranch boundary** - part of a larger linear earthwork, continuing to north and south, with a total length of c8km. See **(VI)**.

(VI) Crossing of ancient ways: a S-N route crossed the E-W line of the Harrow Way, just north of Quarley Hill. As a long, linear earthwork, it came up from Danebury Hillfort, continued northwards over Cholderton Hill and Thruxton Hill, to Sidbury Hill. Its continuation then branched west to join the Great Ridgeway, and east along the North Hampshire Ridgeway, via Scots Poor, towards the North Downs.

(VII) Iron Age settlement site (BC800-AD42) with pits, linear ditches and a banjo enclosure.

Palaeolithic BC500,000-10001 Mesolithic 10000-4001	Neolithic BC4000-2201	Bronze Age BC2200-801	Iron Age BC800-AD42

Roman AD43-409	Early Med/Saxon AD410-1065	Medieval AD1066-1539	Post-Med AD1540-1900

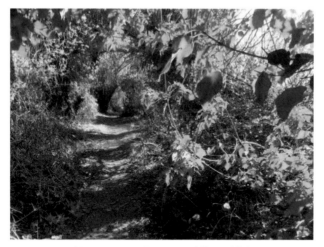

Harrow Way between **(1)** *and* **(2)**

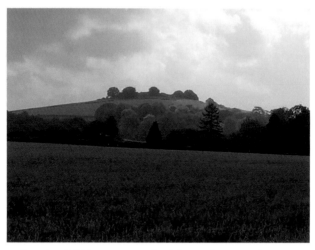

Quarley Hillfort approached from the east, between
(3) *and* **(4)**

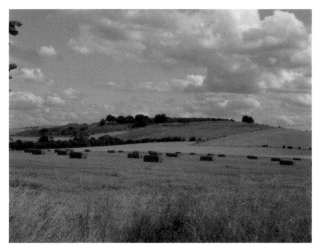

*Northern flanks of Quarley Hillfort, seen from the
Harrow Way*

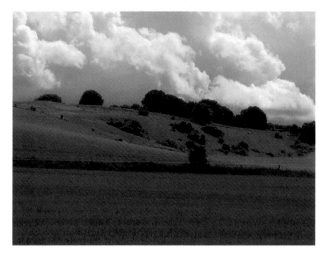

Moody skies above Quarley Hillfort, near **(5)**

76

WALK 5: Setting the Scene

HARROW WAYFARERS in the ROMAN Period (AD43-409)

Following the Roman Invasion in AD43, the fertile farmlands of NW Hampshire became one of the major 'bread baskets' of *Britannia*, with more corn-dryers found here than anywhere else in the country. The rich arable land in turn gave rise to rich native Britons, owning large villas (farm estates) that became increasingly luxurious, reaching their peak in the 4thcentury - some, like Thruxton and Fullerton, with mosaic floors (the former in the British Museum, the latter on display in Andover Museum of the Iron Age). At least five villa sites lie in this area, centred on the market town of *Leucomagus* (East Anton) at the intersection of two major Roman roads: the Portway, linking London and Dorchester, and the Icknield Way, Winchester to Wanborough, near Swindon.

So did the Roman engineers, who sometimes made use of pre-existing Iron Age trackways, incorporate the Harrow Way into their impressive 2000mile road network in *Britannia*? The answer seems to be no, they didn't, at least not in this area. Instead they constructed the Portway, running roughly parallel in places.

If the Harrow Way wasn't being used as an artery of Roman Britain, (to allow the rapid movement of troops and supplies, initially), what, then, was its purpose? A network of local tracks, including the Harrow Way, would link to the main routes, for carrying grain to market, and conveying fine goods, imported from the Continent, to grace the tables and adorn the bodies of the British elite villa owners, aspiring to Roman customs and fashion.

In the shadowy years following Roman withdrawal in AD410, another Romanised (but not at all flashy) Briton, Ambrosius Aurelianus, might have been seen lurking near the Harrow Way, with his band of freedom fighters. Putting up resistance to German mercenaries, he took part in the Battle of *Gualoph/Gualopp*, nearby Wallop, in AD436.

Wealthy villa proprietors? Guerrillas? Could these be our Harrow Wayfarers in the early centuries AD?

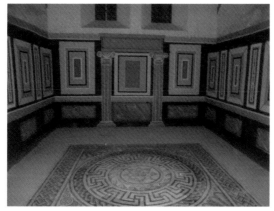

Reconstruction of a Roman villa interior,
courtesy of Butser Ancient Farm

78

WALK 5 ROUTE MAP (see OS Explorer 131)

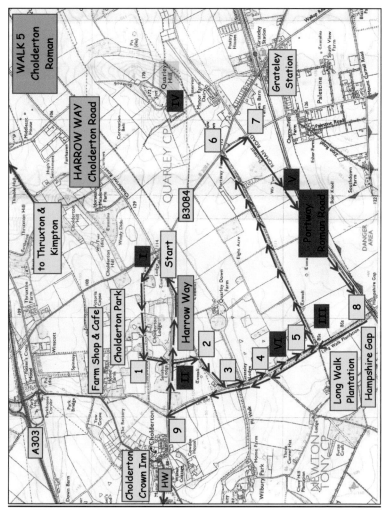

© Crown copyright and database rights 2021 OS Licence 100059949

WALK 5: CHOLDERTON
Focus on the ROMAN Period (AD43-409)

From Harrow Way to Roman road via Bronze Age barrow cemeteries

Portway Roman Road runs roughly parallel to the Harrow Way, west of Andover. Constructed by Vespasian's 2nd Legion, it was part of a major route linking *Londinium* with *Durnovaria* (Dorchester), though the name more precisely refers to the section between *Calleva Atrebatum* (Silchester) and *Sorviodunum* (Old Sarum). The small Romano-British town of *Leucomagus* (East Anton) grew up at the intersection of the Portway (NE-SW) and another important Roman road, running SE-NW. The Roman Army constructed 3200km/2000miles of paved roads in *Britannia* between AD43 and 410.

Practical Information:

Distance:approx **12km/7.5miles. Moderate.**

Parking: Roadside, small lay-by by a Bronze Age tumulus, 2km east of Cholderton, c150m from junction of Cholderton Road and B3084, near lodge at estate entrance.

Refreshments/Toilets: Cholderton Farm Shop and Café, and The Crown Inn, Cholderton, close by. No public toilets.

Terrain: Mainly level tracks, footpaths (may be muddy), bridleways, estate roads, country lanes.

Map:OS Explorer 131 Romsey, Andover & Test Valley.

Grid ref at start point:SU246 423

Best time of year: Winter, when vegetation is low, to view features of Roman road.

About the Walk:

Easy walking along level tracks, footpaths and quiet country lanes on the Cholderton Estate, where creeper-clad flint cottages in the woods, and plaintive cries of peacocks, suggest an air of enchantment - though a very real commitment to biodiversity by the landowner is equally apparent. From an extensive Bronze Age barrow cemetery by the Harrow Way, the walk heads south through an ancient landscape to an impressive 2.2km stretch of Portway Roman Road, with the agger (see below) clearly visible. With thanks to the landowner of Cholderton Estate.

Highlights from the Roman Period:

>long stretch of Portway Roman Road
>agger (ridge of Roman road) clearly visible
>decorated Samian bowl and intaglio (see Glossary) from nearby Kimpton Villa on display in Andover Museum of the Iron Age

Highlights from other periods:
>two Bronze Age barrow cemeteries, including bowl and disc barrows
>Bronze Age hoard findspot – location withheld, but finds, including a socketed axe and palstave (type of axe), can be viewed in Andover Museum
>19th century estate and park

Imagine the Scene in the Roman Period:

On the Harrow Way, follow in the footsteps of Quintus Natalius Natalinus (Footnote i), the highly-Romanised owner of nearby Thruxton Villa, who plans to entertain his friends from neighbouring Kimpton. Quintus is keen to show

81

off his newly-laid mosaic floor, and to admire, in return, their recently-acquired sophisticated item - a decorated Samian bowl, red, glossy and highly-desirable, imported from Gaul. His friend from Kimpton will doubtless be flaunting his flashy *intaglio*, as usual.

Along the Portway, watch for flashes of sunlight on legionary helmets.

At the parking place by the **Harrow Way**, c**150m** from the junction with the B3084, pause to enjoy the close proximity of a large **Bronze Age** bowl barrow (see *Glossary*), the surrounding ditch of which once lay under your car. You have stepped straight into a **4000 year old barrow cemetery**, lying beside the ancient trackway, so take a few moments to look around. Across the road among the trees another burial mound can be made out.

START: Near the junction with the B3084, follow the **footpath sign pointing NW along a track** into Cholderton Park, passing between the brick piles marking the park entrance. **Andover Lodge** on your right, flint-rendered and half-overgrown with ivy, has an almost fairytale feel. All this area is a **Bronze Age barrow cemetery (I)**. A few steps beyond the lodge, look over the metal gate on the left, and you can clearly see a low burial mound, topped with a solitary beech, about 100m into the field, and another further over to the right. The field to the right of the track has two more tumuli, though difficult to see if the grass is high, as they are low. The one nearest the lodge has twin conifers growing out of the left end; the other, by the blue henhouse, is most interesting (see (I)). Where the track bends to the left, look out for another among the trees on the left (please remember that they are all on private land, and should be viewed only from the public right of way). Having rounded the bend, continue westwards along the track lined with neat, silver-barked trees, keeping your head turned to the left for more barrow-spotting. You pass **Cholderton Park House,** built c1800 (marked as Lodge on OS map) on the left, with its range of outbuildings. Look out for your first peacock, stalking sedately through the grounds. Continue **straight ahead** along the track.

(1) When **the track bends sharply to the left,** by a footpath signpost, with **Kingsettle Stud** on the right, a **stable complex with coach houses** built c1900, follow the track round to the **LEFT** down a pretty parkland avenue. This will take you past **Salisbury Lodge** on the right, (again that dream-like quality, if the peacocks are in residence), to the road. This is the **Harrow Way** again. Before crossing the road, see if you can spot Quintus Natalius Natalinus hurrying home, ready to welcome his guests (see 'Imagine the Scene'). **Cross the road with care** and head down the **track** opposite, past Flint Cottage on the right, then **Laundry Cottages.** Beyond a barn on the right lies Laundry Field (II) on private land.

Continue the short distance to the end of the track.

(2) At the quiet **country lane** turn **RIGHT**. After approx **100m**, look for the remains of a tree-topped **Bronze Age** barrow on the right, adjacent to the lane, with another behind in the trees. Continue along the lane to a **T-junction.**

(3) Turn **LEFT** at this junction, signed 'No Through Road', to head southwards along the lane, which shortly becomes a cobbled flint-and-dirt **track** by Grateley Lodge. Follow this **byway** straight ahead (noting a sign 'Hampshire Gap 1mile') down into the dip, which may be muddy. Just beyond an open meadow on your left, with views of Quarley Hill in the distance, watch for a 'Restricted Byway' sign to the right, and a **public footpath** straight ahead.

(4) Go **STRAIGHT AHEAD** along the **footpath** through a broad belt of woodland for approx **800m** until you reach a **crossing of tracks.**

(5) At this crossing, **turn LEFT** to leave Long Walk Plantation and head NE, following the **grassy track** along the **left edge of the field**. Shortly after leaving Long Walk Plantation, a barrow may be visible among the beeches on your left, viewable from the public footpath. On the right is the site of an extensive **Bronze Age** barrow cemetery, including cremation burials (III). Though the tumuli have been ploughed out, a slight rise in the ground may just be visible, in the right light conditions. At an unspecified location between here and the B3084 ahead, a Bronze Age socketed spearhead was found in 1926. This was clearly an important landscape long before the Romans arrived. The grassy track you are following runs parallel to Portway Roman Road, which lies approx 500m away to your right. Follow the left edge of several fields, keeping an eye open for deer. At the time of writing, a line of nine glided silently across the track ahead, the last one pure white. Another magical moment. Carry straight on, past Portway Farm, with a good view of Quarley Iron Age Hillfort (IV) ahead (see Walk 4), and go down the farm track to the main road.

(6)Just before the B3084, turn RIGHT along a secluded footpath, blackthorn and may blossom in season, eventually emerging at the corner of a country lane, with a metal barrier on the right. This marks the start of the Portway.

(7)After emerging from the sheltered footpath, turn RIGHT and go round the barrier to take your first steps along the Portway, with a magnificent 2.2km of Roman road ahead. Follow the bridleway, a flint-and-chalk track, as it undulates gently over down-land, heading SW, the fields on either side concealing a wealth of archaeology. Enjoy the feeling of openness and expanse, imagining, perhaps, that you are walking in the footsteps of those Roman legionaries, pressing on towards *Sorviodunum* (see 'Imagine the Scene'). This is open country, with hedges scarce or low, so it can be exposed in winter. Just over the crest of the rise, beyond the derelict water tower on the left, a well-preserved section of *agger* (V) (see photo p90) stretches away to the horizon, from Quarley Hill behind you to the Hampshire Gap ahead. Take time to savour this special experience and to notice the details. The central track, plus the grassy verges, form the *agger*, raised above the surrounding land. The central track is slightly lower than the verges due to centuries of use. The flanking ditches have either been lost, or are included in this over-all width (c10-12m). See line drawing p90. In due course, the Portway runs side by side with the railway, screened by a belt of tall pines. When the grassy track ends, continue straight ahead along a **woodland footpath**, until you come to an overgrown **railway bridge** on your left – the **Hampshire Gap**.

(8) Leave the Roman legionaries to continue their march towards *Sorviodunum*, turning **RIGHT** here to leave the Portway and take a **footpath** (may be muddy) through **Long Walk Plantation**. The pale trunks of coppiced hazel, along with the silence, might suggest an enchanted forest to the fanciful mind. If you come to a fork in the footpath, take either branch, as they meet up again shortly. Continue **STRAIGHT AHEAD,** passing **(5)** where you left Long Walk Plantation earlier. Where the belt of trees thickens into a copse, this is Quarley

Park Wood **(VI)**. Carry on for several hundred metres, passing Grateley Lodge, until you reach **(3)** again. For the shortest return route, and the least traffic, you can turn **RIGHT** here and follow the quiet country lane all the way back to your vehicle. If, however, you prefer to walk along the Harrow Way (though a busier road) and take in some refreshment, take the **LEFT FORK** at **(3)**, which will lead you in approx **500m** to the **Cholderton Road**, where you are back on the Harrow Way, at **(9)** on the map.

(9)Refreshments: One option is to continue straight ahead for approx **600m** to the **Cholderton Farm Shop and Café** (well worth a visit), or turn left down the road (a path runs adjacent) into Cholderton, to **The Crown Inn** (visit websites).

To complete the walk and enjoy the **Harrow Way,** simply turn **RIGHT** at point **(9)** and head back eastwards along the road to your car, perhaps keeping an eye open for Ambrosius Aurelianus and his band of British freedom fighters (see *Harrow Wayfarers* p77).

Footnote i: The name Quintus Natalius Natalinus was found inscribed on a section of mosaic pavement – the villa owner, or, possibly, the mosaic craftsman. The author has used the former interpretation. (Henig, M. & Soffe, G. The Thruxton Roman Villa and its Mosaic Pavement. See References and Sources p157).

HISTORICAL and ARCHAEOLOGICAL NOTES
(multi-period)

Visits to Andover Museum of the Iron Age, the Willis Museum, Basingstoke, Butser Ancient Farm and the British Museum are highly recommended.

(I) Bronze Age barrow cemetery (BC2200-801): the fields to right and left are the site of at least 14 Bronze Age round barrows, some still visible. Most are **bowl** barrows, though the one mutilated by the blue chicken run shows evidence of having a **disc** barrow superimposed. *See Glossary.*

(II) Laundry Field, a Mid-Late Bronze Age settlement (BC1600-1201): an impressive array of finds is on display in the Museum of the Iron Age, Andover.

(III) Bronze Age barrow cemetery, including cremation burials (BC2200-801): a **disc** barrow revealed a central, primary, cremation burial with a cist (see *Glossary*), accompanied by grave goods. Further cremations were discovered close by, one under an inverted urn. This practice of urn inversion may have been to prevent the spirit of the deceased from escaping. Burnt bone was also found on the surface of the field at the barrow site. A **Bronze Age socketed spearhead**, found in 1926, was loaned to The Salisbury Museum in the 1950s, but subsequently stolen. Good examples of cremation urns and socketed spearheads are on display in the museums in Andover and Basingstoke.

(IV) Quarley Hill: it is thought that Quarley Hill and Cottington Hill, south of Kingsclere, may have been the two prominent landmarks used by Roman surveyors to lay out the straight line of the Portway. From the summit of Quarley Hill, Old Sarum can be seen.

(V) *Agger:* central raised surface of a Roman road, flanked by drainage ditches. A Roman road occupied a wide strip of land, bounded by shallow ditches, varying in width from 25.5m to 100m. In the centre, a **paved carriageway** was constructed, after stripping off the topsoil, on a **substantial raised ridge (agger),** typically 5-8m in width, sometimes more, and up to 1.8m in height, though usually less. The two strips of ground between the *agger* and the boundary ditches, were also used by pedestrians and animals.

(VI) Quarley Park Wood: this extensive woodland was once associated with a large house and gardens. Grateley Lodge (not the smaller lodge that you pass) was described in the Quarley Parish Apportionments of 1840 as a 'pleasure ground'.

Palaeolithic BC500,000-10001 Mesolithic 10000-4001	Neolithic BC4000-2201	Bronze Age BC2200-801	Iron Age BC800-AD42

Roman AD43-409	Early Med/Saxon AD410-1065	Medieval AD1066-1539	Post-Med AD1540-1900

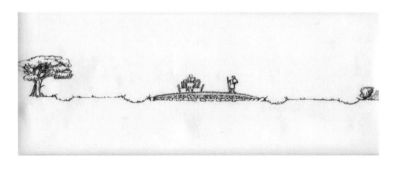

*Raised ridge (agger) of Roman road with flanking ditches.
Line drawing courtesy of David Hopkins*

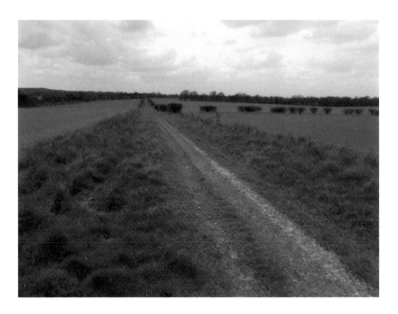

*Portway Roman Road between (7) and (8), looking SW.
Central track and grassy verges form ridge of agger, c10-12m
in width, possibly incorporating former flanking ditches, and
raised above surrounding land*

WALK 6: Setting the Scene
HARROW WAYFARERS in the
EARLY MEDIEVAL (ANGLO-SAXON) Period
(AD410-1065)
Along with drovers, shepherds, farmers, millers
and corn merchants, who else would have been
using the 'Hoare Way' at this time?

Around AD650, a sombre group of mourners might
have been seen making its way along the Harrow
Way to Portway cemetery. A much-loved mother
and wife was being buried, accompanied by her
treasured objects – a knife, bracelet and brooches
– near a man's grave containing a spearhead, shield
and knife (see Andover Museum). These were
pagan burials, but a new religion was already
starting to supplant the old beliefs.

A significant triumph of Christianity over paganism
came in the reign of Ethelred II (r.978-1013 and
1014-16). Despite King Alfred's victory over the
Vikings a century earlier, the pesky pagan
Norsemen were still a nuisance, sailing their
longships up the Test. But at last, in AD994, Olaf
Tryggvason agreed to be converted to Christianity,
in the church at Andover.

Meanwhile, decidedly unholy deeds were taking
place at Weyhill, where large numbers of young
men were being hanged or decapitated, in the
largest Saxon execution site in the country (where
Aldi now stands). As a grisly warning to those

entering the Hundred (see *Glossary*), even minor crimes were punishable by execution – a legacy of Athelstan's Code of Laws, drawn up at nearby Grateley.

Rather unfairly, perhaps, for those petty thieves, a king had got away, quite literally, with murder, several decades earlier. In Harewood Forest, King Edgar had treacherously murdered his earl Ethelwold, who had deceived the king and kept the latter's betrothed for himself. In a strange twist of fate, the Lady Elfthryth, after founding abbeys at Amesbury and Wherwell, to atone for her complicity in this (and another) murder, tumbled into the Test and was drowned.

Whilst we may meet only the ghost of Lady Elfthryth, we will come face to face with another Anglo-Saxon lady, mysterious but clearly of some importance, in All Hallows Church, Whitchurch.

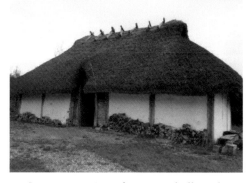

Reconstruction of a Saxon hall, with thanks to Butser Ancient Farm

WALK 6 ROUTE MAP (see OS Explorer 144)

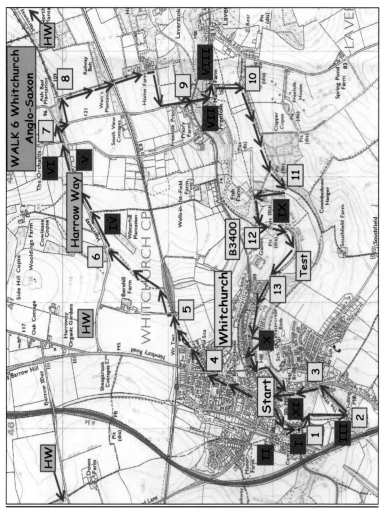

© Crown copyright and database rights 2021 OS Licence 100059949

WALK 6: WHITCHURCH
Focus on the EARLY MEDIEVAL
(ANGLO-SAXON) Period (AD410-1065)

From Harrow Way to Domesday mills and a mysterious Anglo-Saxon lady

Palaeolithic tools, Neolithic pits, Iron Age occupation and a Roman cemetery have all been found in the Whitchurch area, but Hampshire's smallest town is Anglo-Saxon in origin. In AD909 the manor of *Witcerce* ('White Church') was given by Edward the Elder to the monks of Winchester Cathedral. A thriving wool town in the Middle Ages, with a working mill (grain, wool or paper) every half mile, it may also have been the scene of a battle against the Danes in the 10[th]century.

Practical Information:
Distance:approx **11km/6.8miles. Moderate.**
Parking: Free car parks in Bell St and Church St.
Refreshments/Toilets: Choice of pubs and tea shops. Public toilets in Bell Street car park.
Terrain: Pavements, country lanes, tracks, footpaths (may be muddy). One stile, with adjacent gate. Some undulation. Take care when close to water. Dogs on lead, where indicated.
Map:OS Explorer 144 Basingstoke, Alton & Whitchurch.
Grid ref at start point:SU462 481
Best time of year: Any DRY time of year. **Bulls:** occasional signs may indicate presence of a bull, but the Mill Trail is a popular walking route, paths are generally close to field edges, and seasoned ramblers recall no sightings.

94

About the Walk:

This figure-of-eight walk, some of which is along the Mill Trail, starts in the heart of Whitchurch, where the Early Medieval origins of the small town can still be felt, with mills on the site of those listed in the Domesday Survey of 1086 adding picturesque charm by the clear waters of the River Test. A visit to All Hallows Church and its Saxon lady is recommended (check website). Pavements, tracks and footpaths (can be muddy) lead the walker north to join the Harrow Way, a quiet country road, before returning to the valley, and a visit to a further delightful little church with ancient origins at Freefolk. There is a choice of routes for the return to Whitchurch, where a cup of tea beside the mill race at the Silk Mill provides a fitting end for this riverside ramble.

Highlights from the Early Medieval Period:
>church with Anglo-Saxon origins
>fragment of an Anglo-Saxon grave cover with an interesting history
>riverside mills with pre-Conquest roots

Highlights from other periods:
>White Hart coaching inn, with parts dating from the 15thcentury
>famous Silk Mill, still in manufacturing use
>Bere Mill, a former 18thcentury paper mill, once producing the earliest notes for the Bank of England

Imagine the Scene in the Early Medieval Period: From the high ground to the north of Whitchurch, follow in the footsteps of Saxon farmers, still using the ridgeways, much as their forebears had done for centuries, before returning to their thatched, timber-framed, cob or turf dwellings down in the river valley. In the Late Anglo-Saxon period, a string of villages, including Whitchurch, Overton and Andover, grew up along the north bank of the Test, reached from the Harrow Way. And so our weary Saxon Harrow Wayfarers might have ended the day round the fire, earthenware tankard made from grass-tempered clay in hand, sipping beer and relaxing, not unlike their present-day counterparts in the White Hart – save for developments in beer mug manufacture!

START: The walk starts at the mini-roundabout in the centre of town, where five roads meet. Head SW along **Church Street** for approx **300m** to the Church of All Hallows (I) on the corner, where you will make the acquaintance of our mysterious Anglo-Saxon lady. Check website for opening times, as a visit is definitely recommended, but if not possible, see photo of Frithburga's grave cover p108. Before leaving, it is worth reflecting that, whilst the origins of the church are Early Medieval, evidence of much older occupation lies close by, where Neolithic pits (II) were found near Manor Farm.

(1) Leaving the church, cross the road **WITH GREAT CARE** and take the footpath directly opposite, near the corner, to the left of St Cross House, which leads between brick walls and through a wooden gate down to the River Test. You are on a public footpath across private land owned by the Fulling Mill, and must respect the requirements specified on the plaque above the bench on the left.   Turn **RIGHT** along the riverbank (path may be muddy), taking time to enjoy the tranquil scene, until you reach the first of today's four mills, the Fulling Mill (III), now a private house.   Cross the bridge in front of the mill.

(2) As you step off the bridge, turn immediately **LEFT** (ignore the yellow footpath arrow pointing ahead) and follow the **lane,** with its line of picturesque cottages, (the pink thatched one dating from the 17[th]century, with later additions). Over in the field on the left, an old granary (on nine staddle stones, with a half-hipped roof) comes into view, at the foot of tall poplars.

(3) When this lane – The Weir - reaches the main road, Winchester Street, bear **LEFT** along the pavement, back to the mini-roundabout, to complete the initial loop. Take a moment to admire the White Hart Hotel, an 18[th]century coaching inn (though parts may date to the 15[th]century) on the corner of Newbury Street and London Street. Keeping the White Hart on your right, head north up **Newbury Street**, where numbers 5 and 7 were, respectively, a **Medieval shop and shopping parade** (AD1490-1535). Number 5 is now an attractive tea room – Denning's – named after former Whitchurch resident Lord Denning, Master of the Rolls. Other historic houses in Newbury Street date to the 17thand 18thcenturies, and the 'Tudor House' at number 31 to the 16th.

(4) Continue for approx **600m** up the hill, past Kings Walk on the right, then take the **next turning on the right, Dances Lane,** shortly forking **LEFT** to keep on Dances Lane. Pass the Police Station on the right, into Burgage (see *Glossary*) Field 1-4, until the tarmac road ends and a short track leads to a **metal gate** ahead. Go through the gate into a field, site of a **Medieval Deer Park, owned by the Prior of St Swithuns, Winchester** (AD1332). Bear **LEFT,** following the perimeter of the field to the corner, then round to the **RIGHT**, down the slope, with the railway cutting on your left, to a metal gate at the bottom of the field. The field ahead is the site of an **Iron Age or Romano-British settlement enclosure** (BC800-AD409) visible only as cropmarks on aerial photographs.

(5) Go through **two metal gates**, before turning immediately **LEFT** to pass under the **railway bridge**. Immediately after the bridge, turn **RIGHT** through another gate, following the footpath sign displayed on the gate entrance to Berehill Farm. Go down the **grassy track**, with the railway embankment on your right, then at the foot of the slope, follow the hedge round to the **LEFT** along the lower edge of the field, with a drainage ditch on your right (heed the signs for 'deep water'). Keep on this grassy track as it wends its way along by the blackthorn hedge, (snowy white blossom in early spring, sloes in late summer), until you eventually emerge onto a country road – the **Harrow Way.**

(6)Turn **RIGHT** to follow the prehistoric **Harrow Way** for approx **1.2km** as it undulates north-eastwards along a quiet, pleasant country lane, with views to the north, past the entrance to Wooldings Vineyard. Over to the right, just NE of Winterhill Plantation, is evidence of prehistoric activity (IV) and to the left also, in the grounds of Wooldings Farm. Behind Wooldings Cottages lies another prehistoric site (V). Note that, for most of this stretch, the **Harrow Way**, although a ridgeway, lies just off the crest of the ridge, along a terrace on its northern flank. Look for signs of the old drove road, where the modern tarmac strip is flanked by broad grassy verges, separated from surrounding farmland by low banks topped with trees or hedges, the whole terrace being up to approx 10m in width (see photo p110). **Go past** a road leading off to the right, almost **opposite the entrance to Harroway House**, with its impressive sweep of drive leading to an attractive building nestling into the landscape. Just to the left of the house lies **The Orchards (VI)**. Carry on along the road until you reach **Twinley Lane** on the right.

(7) Turn **RIGHT** here up Twinley Lane for a short distance, until you come to a **byway** on the left, and a sign showing cars prohibited Nov – May. This **green lane** is the continuation of the **Harrow Way** eastwards, and extends all the way beyond Overton (see Linear Walk p145). Leave Twinley Lane here and turn **LEFT** to follow the **Harrow Way** along this **byway**, and continue for a couple of hundred metres, noting the grand old yew trees (a sign of antiquity) and an abundance of sloes in season (good news for gin lovers).

(8) After approx **200m**, take the **FIRST TURNING to the right,** (vehicle barriers may be either on or by the **Harrow Way**). Leave the HW here, accompanied, perhaps, by those Anglo-Saxon farmers, making their way down into the valley (see 'Imagine the Scene'). Follow the sheltered **footpath**, in its green tunnel, up to the crest of the ridge, again noting that the ancient ridgeway behind you runs a couple of hundred metres below the crest.   Once over the top, you begin a long, gradual descent towards the valley floor.   The footpath becomes an **unsurfaced track** after a water tower on the right, and low-growing elm and hazel offer welcome shelter from the south-westerlies.   Continue over the **railway bridge**, eventually reaching cottages on the left, where the lane becomes surfaced, passing on your left the tumbledown outbuildings of **Home Farm**. The lane makes a sharp bend to the **right** by North Lodge – follow it round, then down to join another road at a **T-junction**. At the T-junction turn **LEFT** and carry on down the road between (impressively high) banks until **Watch Lane** (the road you are on) emerges onto the **B3400**, by a long terrace of thatched houses on the left – Manor Cottages, the longest run of thatched cottages in the country, built in 1939 by Portals Paper Mill (see Walk 8 Note III) as homes for mill workers.

(9) At this point you have a choice. For the quickest route to St Nicholas' Church, turn LEFT along the main road for approx 150m, then cross the road WITH GREAT CARE to follow the sign to the church. If, however, you have enough time, and want to get a feel for the riverside Medieval settlement of Freefolk (VII), where Domesday mentions a mill, proceed as follows. Cross the B3400 **WITH GREAT CARE** and follow the **track** ahead for a few metres, then turn **LEFT** into a poplar grove, following the footpath/Mill Trail sign. Look to your left, and you can just make out a well house and a spring with a lion head spout, in the wall backing onto the main road - all that remain of a riverside garden dating from 1870. Continue over **two wooden footbridges** then follow the footpath over a **weir**. Cross this with care (it is a very short distance, approx 1.5m), enjoying the watery scene. The footpath leads you through a **wooden gate**, along the side of a field, where there may be electric fences seemingly barring the way (read the instructions carefully). Continue through another **wooden gate**, across a field, then round to the **left** in front of a brick-and-flint cottage with an interesting chimney, and through a **wooden gate with yellow arrow** onto a lane. Turn **LEFT** and follow the lane a short distance towards the **little white church** ahead, noting, in the field on your left, uneven ground that may be a Medieval, or later, moated site (1066-1900). In this tranquil corner, time seems to have stood still. The small, single cell church, with its bell-cote, nestles between Manor Farmhouse and the Priesthouse (see VIII), with the river to the north, and open fields to the south. Go through the gate in the thick yew hedge on the right, and enjoy your visit to this special place – the Church of St Nicholas (VIII).

Leaving the church behind you, retrace your steps back up the **track,** heading away from the main road, continuing past the gate where you emerged onto the lane, round a slight bend to the right (ignoring a wooden gate with a fingerpost on the left) and on up a **long, tree-lined avenue,** with a **footpath signpost with yellow arrow/s** at the top of the slope.

(10)At **the top of the slope,** take the **RIGHT** fork, which leads you onto a **grassy track** running all the way along **the top of the field.** Keep the belt of trees on your left, and the electric fence (at time of writing) on your right. Enjoy the views down into the valley, with the **Harrow Way** on the northern horizon. Keep **STRAIGHT ON** along the top of the field for approx **800m**, keeping the electric fence on your right, until you reach the end of the field. Look carefully for a **wooden gate** in the corner, leading into the next field. If there should happen to be a bull in this field, keep close to the fence. As mentioned earlier, this is a popular, and well-used, public right of way. Following the top edge of the field, go over the crest and down the slope to a **wooden gate**.

(11) To return to Whitchurch by the most direct route, you can go through the wooden gate and follow the clearly-signed Mill Trail all the way back to the town, emerging near Town Mill (see (X) below). Alternatively, to get a good view of the second mill of the day, and to follow the north bank of the river, where the Saxon settlement is likely to have been, proceed as follows. Just **before** the wooden gate, turn **RIGHT** down the slope, through a gap in the fence at the bottom, turning **RIGHT** along the track towards Bere Mill **(IX),** now a private house, with a view of its stunning waterside garden (the mill race) on your left. Go through a **gate**, or over the adjacent **stile,** along by a wall, and round to the front of the property, where a **bridge** just beyond Bere Mill Butchery (selling local free range produce and well worth a visit, if you have room in your backpack) affords the best view of Bere Mill, where restoration may still be taking place after a disastrous fire in 2018. It is still a beautiful spot, and the gardens are sometimes open to the public as part of the National Gardens Scheme – check website for information. **Cross the bridge**, enjoying the views, and head towards the main road along the lane for approx **200m.**

(12) Approx **200m** beyond the bridge, watch carefully for a **wooden gate** on the left. Leave the lane here and turn **LEFT** through the wooden gate (dogs on lead) into a field, maybe with sheep for company, then **STRAIGHT ACROSS**, heading for a **gate** on the far side. From here the footpath (still the Mill Trail) back to Whitchurch is clearly signed, easy to follow (though may be muddy), and separated from any bovine inhabitants of the field. On your left, the river flows quietly, past old mossy willows. Although Anglo-Saxon dwellings, being made of timber, leave little trace, you might like to imagine small thatched huts dotting the north bank, perhaps clustered round a larger hall (see photo in *Harrow Wayfarers* p91).

(13) Continue until you eventually emerge onto a road in a residential area of the town, by a green (at time of writing) chalet-style bungalow. After approx **200m,** at **The Green**, fork **LEFT**, then almost immediately **LEFT** again, by **Pound Meadow**, along a narrow tarmac path between garden fences, leading you eventually to the river and **Town Mill (X)**, the third of today's four mills. To complete the remaining distance to the fourth and final mill, turn **RIGHT** along Town Mill Lane, by a branch of the river, for the short distance to the **main road (London Street).** Turn **LEFT** here for approx **100m,** then **LEFT** again down **Test Road,** which will lead you in due course to **Winchester Street**, almost opposite the Silk Mill (XI), the last mill of the day, and the only one still in working order. Time for tea and cake by the mill race, with ducks for company this time, before heading back up Winchester Street to the mini-roundabout, and your vehicle.

HISTORICAL and ARCHAEOLOGICAL NOTES
(multi-period)
Visits to Andover Museum of the Iron Age, and to Butser Ancient Farm, are recommended.
(I) Church of All Hallows: the 'White Church' may indeed have been white, made of chalk or cob, until the Normans built over it in stone. The pre-Conquest local church lay within the grounds of the manor house, to serve the lord or thegn (see *Glossary*). Nothing remains of this, but Manor Farm, marked on the OS map to the NW of the church, dates from 1450-1525 and was held by St Swithun's Priory. In 1132, the church and all its property were given by Bishop Henri de Blois to St Cross Hospital, Winchester. **Saxon grave cover of Frithburga:** a wonderful relic of the 10[th]century has survived, via a somewhat tortuous route. A stone fragment of a grave cover can be seen near the lectern or pulpit (it is still on the move!), showing the head of Christ, and

commemorating Frithburga, clearly a lady of some standing in the community, possibly a nun from Wherwell Abbey. The stone was found lodged in the walls of the Norman church, then, in the 19th century, used as a step for a bell ringer! A helpful leaflet in the church gives further information.

(II) Neolithic pits (BC4000-2201): seven pits containing sherds of Neolithic pottery - Fengate ware and Grooved ware (see *Glossary* 'Neolithic Pottery') - and some charred hazelnut shells, were found in the vicinity of Manor Farm.

(III) Fulling Mill: 18th century watermill, on the site of one mentioned in Domesday (1086), built as a fulling mill (see *Glossary*), later used as a corn mill in the 19th century.

(IV) Prehistoric trackways (BC4000-AD42) or field boundaries are visible as cropmarks on aerial photographs, both to the south and north of the Harrow Way.

(V) Bronze Age barrow (BC2200-801) visible as cropmarks on aerial photographs.

(VI) The Orchards: farmhouse first documented in AD1327 as *Atte Norcharde*, home of Robert Atte Norcharde.

(VII) Freefolk: *Frigefole* is first recorded in Domesday (1086) as a village and a mill. The name is believed to mean 'The Free Folk' or 'Freeholders', ie a settlement outside the feudal system.

(VIII) Church of St Nicholas: Late Medieval single cell church, built on the site of an 11th century building. The walls may date to the

13th century, but the whole appears to be 15th century, restored 1703. It contains fragments of 17th century wall paintings, and, on the north wall of the nave, a depiction of St Christopher, dating to the early 15th century. The tomb monument of Sir Richard Powlett (1624) is surrounded by a wrought-iron rail. Adjacent to the church lies the **Priesthouse,** dating to 1700.

(IX) Bere Mill: Henry Portal, a Huguenot refugee, took over the lease of Bere Mill in the early 18th century, and, in 1724, began producing the earliest monetary notes for the Bank of England. Production subsequently transferred to Laverstoke Mill (now Bombay Sapphire Distillery), then to its present site, Overton Mill (see Walk 8 Note III).

(X) Town Mill: a watermill in the 18th century, a corn mill in the 19th, and recently converted to a private dwelling. An iron waterwheel has been remounted at the southern end of the house.

(XI) Silk Mill: Domesday (1086) records a probable corn mill on this site. The present Silk Mill dates from 1800, when it was used initially as a fulling mill, and by the 1830s a silk mill with over 100 employees, including children. Prestigious fabrics were produced here, including ottoman silk for legal gowns. Owned by the Hampshire Buildings Preservation Trust, leased to the Whitchurch Silk Mill Trust, it is the last working mill of its kind in S England, managed as a working museum, where silk is woven for interiors, fashion and theatrical costumes.

107

Palaeolithic BC500,000-10001 Mesolithic 10000-4001	Neolithic BC4000-2201	Bronze Age BC2200-801	Iron Age BC800-AD42

Roman AD43-409	Early Med/Saxon AD410-1065	Medieval AD1066-1539	Post-Med AD1540-1900

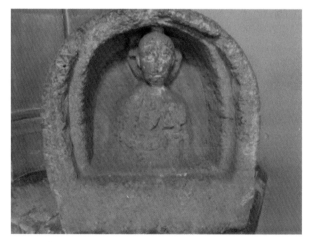

10thcentury Saxon grave cover commemorating Frithburga (I) in All Hallows Church, Whitchurch

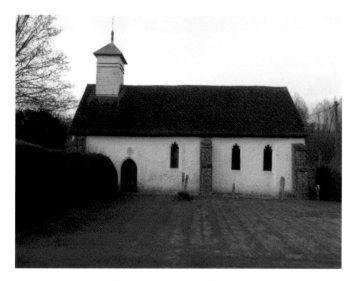

St Nicholas' Church, Freefolk (VIII)

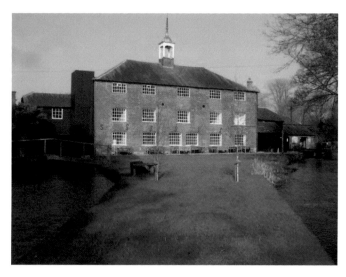

Whitchurch Silk Mill (XI)

109

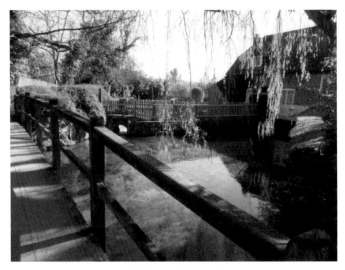

Fulling Mill (III)

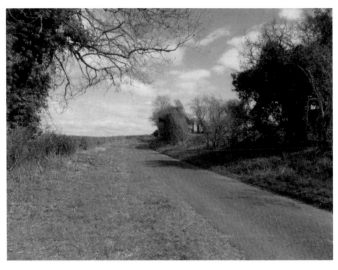

Harrow Way – old drove road – near **(6)**

110

WALK 7: Setting the Scene

HARROW WAYFARERS in the MEDIEVAL Period (AD1066-1539)

Wool was a valuable commodity in the Middle Ages, and the fleecy providers thereof were often herded great distances to markets and fairs – a former drovers' inn in Stockbridge, reached down a branch track from the Harrow Way, still has a sign in Welsh on the front wall, advertising 'Season's Hay, Rich Grass, Good Ale and Sound Sleep'.

In the Andover area, all drove roads converged on Weyhill. One of England's oldest and most important Medieval fairs, going back at least to the Norman Conquest, the thrice-yearly Weyhill Fair traded at its peak 100,000 sheep a day, as well as cattle in spring and hops in autumn. Wild beasts, curiosities and side shows added entertainment, and the cheese fair allowed an 18[th]century local parson to sample 54 varieties in one day! Labourers could be hired at the Mop Fair, and even wives sold – a certain Betty Duck changed hands for half a crown, perhaps providing the inspiration for Thomas Hardy's sale of Mrs Henchard in *The Mayor of Casterbridge*.

Talking of inspiration, Chaucer, who owned nearby Ramridge House in the 14[th]century, may have spotted prototypes for the drunken miller and worldly Wife of Bath at the Fair. Along with these Canterbury-bound pilgrims, others could have been making their way to St Swithun's shrine in

111

Winchester, rubbing shoulders along the Harrow Way with messengers, musicians, merchants, pedlars, priests, bishops, revenue collectors, travelling justices, ale tasters … and even royalty. King John stayed at the Angel in Andover in 1205, and Henry II had a residence north of Overton.

William I may well have cantered along the summer route of the Harrow Way, on his victory march from Hastings to Winchester in 1066. Two decades later, William's men would have been out covering the length and breadth of the country, collecting detailed information about the land, its use and its inhabitants – down to the last ox and pig. The astonishingly-comprehensive result of this survey was the Domesday Book of 1086.

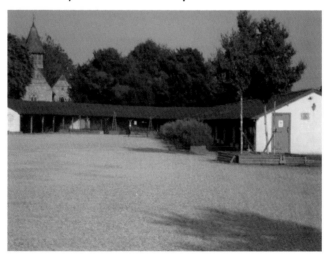

Weyhill Fairground today, where craft centres, studios and a tea room replace Medieval stalls

WALK 7 ROUTE MAP (see OS Explorer 144)

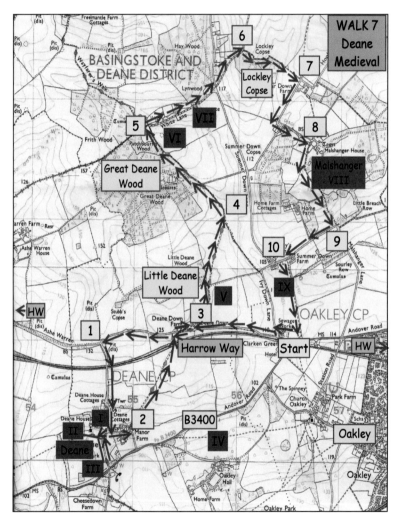

© Crown copyright and database rights 2021 OS Licence 100059949

WALK 7: DEANE and MALSHANGER
Focus on the MEDIEVAL Period (AD1066-1539)

From Harrow Way to a Deserted Medieval Settlement and a Tudor Tower

This walk takes us right back to the time of the Domesday Book in 1086, when William the Conqueror commissioned an exhaustive survey of his recently-conquered kingdom, in order to ascertain the full extent of his wealth and manpower. The walk spans the entire Medieval period, from the 11th century, when Saxon villages were still thriving communities, to the late 15th, by which time many had died, due to the enclosure of common land for the landowner's use. The sheep that had brought prosperity to this area had a human cost.

Practical Information:

Distance: approx **12km/7.5miles. Moderate.**

Parking: At Beach Arms Hotel, if a meal is intended, or on the roadside hard standing in front of the nearby Wastewater Treatment Works.

Refreshments/Toilets: At start/end, Beach Arms Hotel, Clarken Green, just west of Oakley on the B3400. No public toilets.

Terrain: Gently undulating. Footpaths, bridleways and quiet country lanes. Possibly muddy in places, and best avoided after prolonged periods of rain, as springs at Deane can cause extensive flooding. Dogs must be kept under close control where indicated, especially in Malshanger Park.

114

Map:OS Explorer 144 Basingstoke, Alton & Whitchurch.

Grid ref at start point:SU564 510

Best time of year: Any **dry** time of year (see 'Terrain' overleaf). Late winter for the dark outline of bare branches along the Harrow Way, and snowdrops in Deane. Springtime for bluebells in Great Deane Wood. August for strip paths through cornfields. **Bulls:** occasional signs may indicate the presence of a bull, but the Wayfarers' Walk is an official, and popular, long-distance trail.

About the Walk:

A delightful figure-of-eight ramble across rolling farmland and parkland. It starts along the Harrow Way, a busy drove road in the Middle Ages, dips down to explore Deane, before heading northwards along the Wayfarers' Walk (WW) and an old salt route. Footpaths, bridleways (may be muddy) and quiet country lanes lead the walker on, through a Post-Medieval Deer Park, where the silence is broken only by birdsong in the leafy canopy. The atmosphere of Feudal England still lingers in the sleepy hamlets of Deane and Malshanger.

Highlights from the Medieval Period:

>site of a Deserted Medieval Settlement (DMS)

>Tudor Tower

>Tudor Farmhouse: early 16thcentury hall house

Highlights from other periods:

>Roman villa site

>17th/18thcentury Deane House, with Jane Austen associations

>early 19thcentury Malshanger House and Park

Imagine the Scene in the Medieval Period:
In the latter part of the 11thcentury, small ponies might have been seen trotting along the Harrow Way, bearing burly barons to the manorial court in Deane, held in the church, the manor house, or the open air. Collecting information for the Domesday Survey, they would have been preparing to ask detailed questions about the lord of the manor's estate – haw many men, mills, meadows, fishponds, ploughs, hides ... in short, how much money could the demesne (see *Glossary*) add to the king's coffers, and how many men to his army?

Take the B3400 to **Clarken Green**, just west of Oakley, where the railway line crosses the Andover Road/B3400. The Beach Arms Hotel is approx **150m** from a sharp bend under a railway bridge. Turn off the B3400 to head up **Ivy Down Lane**, between the Beach Arms and a garage, signed to Hannington. After approx **150m** you pass under (another) railway bridge, and the Wastewater Treatment Works are on the right. There is hard standing here for parking, but take care not to block the entrance.

START: Immediately beyond the railway bridge on Ivy Down Lane, turn **LEFT** to follow the quiet country road westwards, keeping the railway line on your left. This is the **Harrow Way**. After a rather dull start close to the railway line, it soon begins a gradual ascent, between grand old oaks.

116

Approx **800m** after setting out, just before **Deane Down Farm** on the right, watch for a **wooden footpath signpost and metal gate** on the right, with a green Wayfarers' Walk arrow on one side, indicating the route you will follow later at (3). **Carry on** for approx **150m** along the **Harrow Way**, past Deane Down Farm, watching for the Wayfarers' Walk joining from the left. Look to see if there is a somewhat waggish sign saying 'Entrance to the field is FREE. The BULL will charge later'. If the field has an occupant, you can make an informed decision later! Carry on along the Harrow Way as it continues a gentle rise across farmland - sometimes exposed, sometimes sheltered - with wild flowers in the bank in season. Just beyond the crest of the ridge, approx **2km** after setting out, a **road** runs down to the left, signed **Deane**.

(1) Turn **LEFT** here by a steep bank to leave the **Harrow Way**, following in the footsteps of the **Harrow Wayfarers (see 'Imagine the Scene')**, and head down for a little tour of Deane, documented in the Domesday Book as *Dene,* meaning 'valley'. As you come into the village, bear **RIGHT** then, at the next corner, leave the road and **TURN RIGHT** again, through a **metal gate** beside a white gate, to follow a **paved footpath** along in front of the magnificent 17th/18thcentury mansion, Deane House (I), heading for the **church**. After prolonged rain, springs well up here, flooding the fields and the path to the church, so choose your weather conditions carefully. Beyond Deane House lies the early 19ᵗʰcentury Church of All Saints, on the site of the former Medieval church, of which nothing remains. The nave of the Medieval church may have been the location of the manorial court (see *Glossary*). By the church, go through the metal gate into the field, and follow the footpath along the edge of the field for a few metres. Just beyond the boundary hedge of the graveyard, look to your right, and you may notice that, beyond the fence, the rising ground, dotted with clumps of trees, is uneven (see photo p128). Please be aware that this is on private land, and must be viewed from the footpath. These **grassy mounds** are important indicators: though not spectacular, they tell a powerful story of a Deserted Medieval Settlement (II).

To continue the tour of Deane, return past Deane House to the village road, then turn **RIGHT** to head the short distance down towards the B3400, noting, over to the right, more grassy ridges and terraces - all that remain of the landscaped gardens of Deane Park. You also pass, on the right, the site of the Old Rectory (III), though there is nothing to mark the spot. Retrace steps back up to where the road came down from the Harrow Way. Decision time. If a bull was sighted in the field by the Harrow Way earlier, you can simply retrace your steps up the lane to the Harrow Way, then back to Deane Down Farm. If, however, you wish to take the Wayfarers' Walk across the fields, follow the village lane round to the **RIGHT,** past a row of picturesque thatched cottages, which may date from the 16ᵗʰcentury phase of relocation, when Deane Park was landscaped (see (IV)). The first on the left is Tudor Farmhouse, a thatched four-bay hall house, dated by roof timbers to AD1524. Continue for approx **100m**, past the entrance to Manor Farm on the right, where uneven ground is documented as marking old Medieval boundaries.

(2) Just before the bend, leave the lane and **TURN LEFT** as indicated by a **footpath sign** with the **green WW arrow**. At the end of the short drive, bear **RIGHT** by the wooden gate, following the green arrow along by the fence. Pass behind a corrugated iron outhouse, and you will spot a **wooden gate** at a gap in the hedge ahead. Following the direction indicated by the green and yellow arrows, head **diagonally** across the field in a north-easterly direction along a delightful **strip path** through the crops in summer (wind in the barley, perhaps). Looking back to the SE, you should be able to catch a glimpse of Oakley Hall (IV) beyond the B3400. Continue through a gap in the hedge and across another field, over the **railway bridge** to the edge of the 'bull field', then the short distance back to the road (the Harrow Way). Turn **RIGHT** along the road for approx **100m**, past **Deane Down Farm**. Immediately beyond the outbuildings, watch for the **wooden footpath signpost** with a green WW arrow, on the

119

left, that you noted on the outward journey, by a **metal gate**.

(3) Leave the Harrow Way, and turn **LEFT** through the metal gate, to follow the **Wayfarers' Walk (WW)**. If there is another bull sign here, look carefully to establish the occupant's position, as there is no obvious alternative route. Leaving the road behind you, head **straight up** the left edge of the first field, then **diagonally RIGHT** across the second, following the arrow, to a **metal gate** in the far right corner of the field, at the foot of an oak. Go through the gate and the bushes to emerge into a field. Turn **LEFT** to follow the field edge. Just to the right of the path, in the corner of the field, look for a slightly **raised area** – discernible if you compare it with the flatness of the rest of the field. This is the site of a Roman villa (V). In the corner of the field by the villa site, a track comes in from the right. **Cross the track** to spot a **wooden footpath signpost on the left,** at the corner of **Little Deane Wood,** with a **green WW arrow pointing diagonally right** across the field. Follow this direction, leaving the wood behind you, and enjoying the open views.

(4) At the far side of the field you reach a broad **grassy track** coming up from the right (a continuation of Ivy Down Lane). Turn **LEFT** to follow this pleasant **bridleway,** still the WW, up a gradual rise, with a bank of brambles and bracken on your left, and occasional oaks lining the path.

Continue past **Great Deane Wood**, with its carpet of bluebells in spring, on your left, followed by **Patchbourne Wood**, until you come to the final stretch of hedge-lined bridleway (may be muddy), leading down to a **track across your path**, where the WW carries on ahead, and the track to the left is part of a cycle trail. The field on the right has an interesting findspot **(VI)**.

(5) At this point, leave the Wayfarers' Walk and turn **RIGHT** to follow what quickly becomes a surfaced lane - White Lane **(VII)**, a name often indicative of an old salt route, conveying salt inland from the coast. The primary function of this old salt route now, though, seems to be to provide access to the upmarket houses lining its northern side, some with stables and paddocks. At the **crossroads** with **Hannington Lane** (marked Summer Down Lane on the OS map), where a bench is conveniently situated beside the signpost, cross the road and continue **STRAIGHT AHEAD** up the country lane, as it climbs past more grand houses hidden in the trees on your left.

(6) Approx **500m** beyond the crossroads, as the road bends sharply to the left, watch for a **wooden fingerpost** on the right, at the entrance to a short **gravel track** leading off to the right, blocked very shortly by a **large log**, deliberately placed on its side to prevent vehicular access. Go round the log then follow the footpath round to the **RIGHT** along the edge of the field, keeping the tall hedge/trees on your right. The footpath joins an **unsurfaced track** – follow this round to the **LEFT**, down the slope into the dip, with **Lockley Copse** on your right. After the copse ends, follow the track ahead, with a hedge on the left and a flinty field on the right, until you emerge through an open gate by what looks like a hangar on the left (ignore any footpath signs here) onto a **country lane at a sharp bend**, close to Shear Down Farm, first documented in AD1334.

(7) Turn **RIGHT** here along the quiet road for approx **200m**, then sharp **LEFT** at the corner, past a green space with swings and a simple playground roundabout on the right, and a group of lattice-paned **estate cottages**. Continue uphill past a copse on the right until you come to **Oakley Bowling Club** on your left. An Arcadian whiff of 'Merrie England' hangs in the air in this peaceful corner, with its spreading oaks and chestnuts.

(8) Just beyond **Oakley Bowling Club** on the left, and an enormous yew hedge, turn **RIGHT** along the lane, watching for tantalising glimpses on the left of the octagonal Malshanger Tower, all that remains of the early 16thcentury Tudor Manor, built by an Archbishop of Canterbury (VIII). There is much to enjoy here – quaint Garden Cottage on the left, a mid-19thcentury estate worker's cottage, grassy verges with daffodils in season – followed by a delightful wander down the lane through what was once a Post-Medieval Deer

Park. Keep looking out for the occasional brief view of Malshanger House over to the left, with the tower behind. Enjoy the tall beeches and old yews in the woods, where the modern world feels pleasantly remote. Remember, though, that you are on a public footpath across private land, and dogs must be kept under close control.

(9) You emerge from Malshanger Park by a charming lattice-paned lodge, dated c1869. Turn **RIGHT** here to head along a **country lane,** past the turning to Home Farm on the right, with tall lime trees on either side, until you come to **Summer Down Farm** on the left.

(10)Immediately beyond Summer Down Farm, just as the garden fence ends, watch for a **gap in the hedge on the left,** between two telegraph poles, and an old, ivy-clad wooden footpath signpost. (If you get to a bend in the road and a signpost to Malshanger and Hannington, you have gone too far). Go through the **gap in the hedge** to follow the footpath round to the left, until there is a good view of the front/rear of this attractive brick house, then bear **RIGHT** to follow a **grassy path** along the edge of the field, with **three old oaks** on your left (watch for kestrels in the vicinity). You are very close to a Stone Age findspot (IX). Head back towards the main road and the Wastewater Treatment Works, with a lovely old hedge on your left, interspersed with wild fruit trees, and blossom in season. At the corner of the field bear **RIGHT** along a **permissive footpath** that leads (briefly) past the Sewage Works on the left, back out onto Ivy Down Lane a few steps from your vehicle.

Refreshment may be called for at **Beach Arms Hotel**, the name of which commemorates the rather splendidly-named Right Hon. William Wither Bramston Beach who, at his death in 1901, was Father of the House of Commons.

HISTORICAL and ARCHAEOLOGICAL NOTES (multi-period)
A visit to the Willis Museum in Basingstoke is highly recommended.
(I) Deane House: a beautifully-proportioned country mansion, with views over Deane Park, and a flight of scalloped stone steps descending to sweeping lawns. It was begun in either AD1600 or 1786 (two reliable sources differ). Jane Austen attended dances held here by the Harwoods, and met the dashing Irishman Tom Lefroy (see Walk 8 Note (VI)).
(II) DMS (Deserted Medieval Settlement) (see *Glossary*): the original village lay just to the west of the church, where 'humps and bumps' are the only indicators today of the DMS, where agricultural workers lived, loved, worked and died. In the Middle Ages it was moved to what is now Oakley Park, a short distance SE of Deane, when the new manor of **Hall Place (now Oakley Hall)** was being built (see **(IV)**).

(III) Old Rectory, site of: Jane Austen's father was rector here 1764-68, having been given the living of Deane, as well as Steventon. From 1790-92 it was the home of Jane's close friends Martha and Mary Lloyd and their mother, with Mary in time becoming the second wife of Jane's brother James.

(IV) Re-siting of the Medieval village: in the north of Oakley Park, fieldwork has revealed seven 13th-14thcentury crofts, linked by a sunken pathway, and a small timber farmstead from later 14th-16thcentury occupation. A wide scatter of pottery, including Saxon, was found, along with a sherd of Tudor Green. Although environmental factors such as flooding may have played a part in the relocation of the village, it was probably due to the enclosing of arable land for lucrative sheep farming, which had begun in the 13thcentury. In the late 15thcentury, influential Tudor landowners began buying up the old ecclesiastical estates, in order to enclose them for their own use. In the 16thcentury, the landscaping of Deane Park may also have played a part in the village re-siting, though some documentary sources put this much later.

(V) Roman villa (AD43-409): near the SE corner of Little Deane Wood, a raised area in the corner of the field indicates where the villa once stood. Flints, tile fragments and pottery, including Samian ware (see *Glossary*), have been found in abundance.

(VI) Findspot: Iron Age and Roman pottery (BC800-AD409): two tile fragments from 'White

Lane 1944' seen in the Willis Museum, Basingstoke. The Iron Age pottery includes a bead-rim jar and 'Belgic' platter (a style imported from the Continent by the native Romano-British), which were found in association with Roman pottery and building material. Further south in the same field, **Neolithic flints** were found.

(VII) White Lane: often indicates an old **salt route**, conveying this valuable commodity inland from the coast, from prehistoric times right through to Medieval and later. In the Iron Age, salt was the only food preservative that was reliable all year round, so it is highly likely that some of the Iron Age pottery found just to the south of White Lane (see (VI)) was associated with its transportation.

(VIII) Malshanger Tower, House and Park: at the time of Domesday in 1086, the hides (see *Glossary*) at *Mals(h)anter* (probably denoting the hillside wood of someone called Mal), were in the possession of the Governor of Windsor Castle, ancestor of the baronial house of Windsor. In 1504, the estate was bought by William Wareham, Chancellor of England and Archbishop of Canterbury. **Malshanger House** is a grand early 19thcentury mansion, roughly contemporary with the **Park**.

(IX) Flints findspot, Palaeolithic, Mesolithic, Neolithic (BC500,000-2201): flint implements found in the vicinity of Summer Down Farm, stored in the Willis Museum, Basingstoke, where there is a good display of Stone Age tools.

Palaeolithic BC500,000-10001 Mesolithic 10000-4001	Neolithic BC4000-2201	Bronze Age BC2200-801	Iron Age BC800-AD42

Roman AD43-409	Early Med/Saxon AD410-1065	Medieval AD1066-1539	Post-Med AD1540-1900

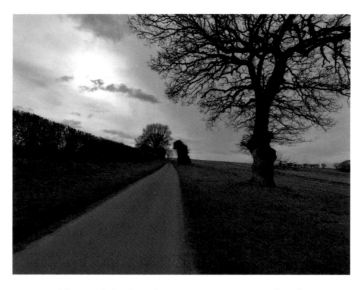

Harrow Way heading west, near start of walk

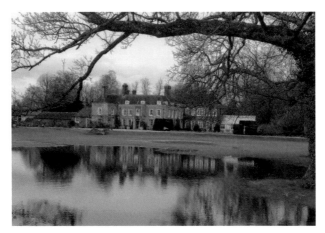

Deane House (I) viewed from public footpath, over flooded lawns

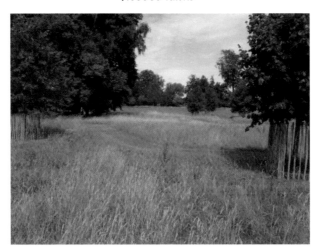

Site of Deserted Medieval Settlement (II) to the west of the church in Deane

WALK 8: Setting the Scene

HARROW WAYFARERS in the POST-MEDIEVAL Period (AD1540-1900)

Wool, water power and Winchester Bishops had all played a part in helping Overton to flourish during the Middle Ages. By the 16[th]century, the village was enjoying a further period of growth and prosperity. With its prime location at the foot of the chalk downs, by the River Test, its economy was based largely on corn and wool (Henry III had granted Overton what was probably the first official sheep fair in 1246). An increasing number of mills were springing up along the river, including corn, fulling (*see Glossary*), and even a silk mill.

In the 16[th]and 17[th]centuries, the Harrow Way was still an important thoroughfare, used by drovers and shepherds, farmers and traders, millers and merchants, and those upholding law and order – constables, bailiffs, beer tasters and reeves (*see Glossary*), as well as the Bishop's steward, officiating at the manorial court held in the courthouse in the town.

But the 18[th]century brought change, with the establishment of Turnpike Trusts (*see Glossary*). Travel was no longer in the slow lane. Thundering through the centre of Overton, at the thrilling speed of 10mph, the London-Exeter stagecoach, carrying mail and passengers, cut the 170mile journey time from four days in the 1720s to 17 hours in 1835. Coaching inns, such as the White

Hart (see *Glossary*) in Andover, Whitchurch and Overton, with their cobbled yards, stables, and welcoming landlords and landladies, provided sustenance to weary passengers and horses, at all hours of the day and night.

The end of a very long era ...
Sadly, this turnpike revolution did indeed toll the knell of ridgeways, principal thoroughfares for millennia, though it didn't supplant them entirely. Shrewd drovers and shepherds still preferred to herd their flocks to market along the green lanes, to avoid the tolls.

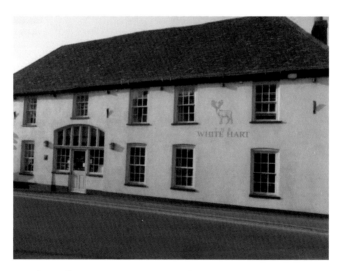

The White Hart, Overton, a former coaching inn (X)

WALK 8 ROUTE MAP (see OS Explorer 144)

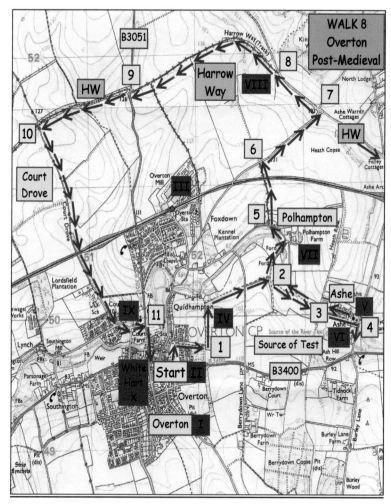

© Crown copyright and database rights 2021 OS Licence 100059949

WALK 8: OVERTON and ASHE
Focus on the POST-MEDIEVAL Period
(AD1540-1900)

From Harrow Way to a historic market town and an old coaching inn

Galloping hooves, the clamour of voices in the stable yard – sounds that would have met weary travellers taking refreshment in the White Hart, Overton, 200 years ago, as the London-Exeter stagecoach rolled in. Up on the Harrow Way, more peaceful, bleating sounds would have prevailed, as they had done for centuries.

Practical Information:

Distance:approx **10.5km/6.5miles. Moderate.**

Parking: Free car park in London Road, at the recycling centre by Turnpike Cottages, about 200m east of the crossroads and traffic lights in the centre of the village, in direction of Basingstoke.

Refreshments/Toilets: Good choice of tea rooms and pubs in Overton, including the White Hart. No public toilets.

Terrain: Quiet country roads, pavements, tracks, footpaths, byways (may be muddy). Some gentle undulation. Dogs must be kept under control.

Map:OS Explorer 144 Basingstoke, Alton & Whitchurch.

Grid ref at start point:SU517 497

Best time of year:A dry summer day, perhaps, as the fields over to Ashe can be boggy. Harrow Way quieter Nov-May, when closed to off-road vehicles. Winter for catkins, summer for wild mint in the Test rivulet.

132

About the Walk:

Leaving Overton, follow footpaths eastwards across farmland and water meadows, past the source of the Test, to the quiet hamlet of Ashe, with its Jane Austen associations. Retrace steps to Polhampton, another Domesday settlement, and head up to the Harrow Way. Stride out along a magnificent stretch of this old drove road, where giant catkins dangle in season, before returning to Overton for refreshment at the historic White Hart, or one of the charming tea rooms.

Highlights from the Post-Medieval Period:

>splendid old coaching inn with a long and interesting history

>drove roads - Harrow Way and Court Drove

>Ashe House, with its literary associations

Highlights from other periods:

>Bishop of Winchester's Medieval palace and courthouse

>Mesolithic and Neolithic flint findspots in abundance

>two hamlets recorded in Domesday Book 1086

Imagine the Scene in the Post-Medieval Period:
From the Harrow Way, follow in the footsteps of 18th century shepherds, herding their woolly charges down to the annual sheep fair in the wide main street of the market town, which had grown up early in the 13th century south of the river, leaving the old Saxon village and church to the north. Follow in daintier footsteps too, with Jane Austen as she visits friends at Ashe House.

START: The walk starts in **Overton (I)**, in the free car park in London Road, approx **200m** east of the crossroads and traffic lights in the centre of the village. From the car park by **Turnpike (II) Cottages** head over into the Community Orchard, adjacent to the car park, along the narrow path, joining a surfaced footpath by the Overton Hill Play Area, and following it round to the right, up the slope. Excavations ahead of this Overton Hill residential development revealed **Iron Age, Roman and Saxon settlements** (BC800-AD1065) - see Walk 3 Note (I). Continue up the slope, crossing a small road, and carry on **STRAIGHT AHEAD** into 'Sheep Field', keeping an eye open for ovine sculptures hiding among the bushes. At the bench near the top of the field, pause to look back over the village, and note the chimneys of **Overton Mill (III)** to the right.

(1) At the very top of this field, make sure you bear **LEFT**, ignoring other footpath signs and arrows. Having turned left at the top of the field, continue down a **grassy track** at the **left edge** of the field, taking a moment to think of older travellers who passed this way long ago (IV). At the corner in the dip, continue round to the **RIGHT**, keeping to the field edge, with an area of scrub on your left. After approx **100m**, leave the line of bushes on your left to head **STRAIGHT ACROSS** the field, along a strip path cut through the crop (see photo p144), aiming for a wooden gate at the far side of the field. In this field, and

134

the next, several more pieces of **Mesolithic struck flint** were found. Go through the **gate** at the far side of the field, cross a narrow lane (**beware cyclists**), through another gate, then **CONTINUE AHEAD** bearing slightly left along another strip path through the field. The quiet hamlet of Polhampton nestles in the hollow on the left, where the young Test, just a stream here, flows quietly through a willow and poplar grove.

(2)You are about to do a short detour to Ashe, with its Post-Medieval associations, before retracing steps to this point. At the far side of the field that you are in, at the foot of the slope, **DON'T** go through the gate by the stile in the corner, but continue **round to the left**, and almost immediately look for a **small footbridge** among the willows on the right, with three yellow arrows. **CROSS** the footbridge ('The Pullinger Family – Footbridge Gate') into a field where sheep may be quietly grazing. **DOGS MUST BE KEPT UNDER CONTROL.** Head **straight across** the water meadow, pausing to admire the young Test on your right (source in next field) where wild mint grows in summer. Aim for a **gate in the hedge** at the far side of the field, towards Ashe.

(3)Go through the gate and a narrow belt of woodland, then **straight ahead** along a **grassy track** by a row of lime trees, with the hamlet of Ashe ahead – *Esse*, meaning 'At the Ash Tree' (Domesday Book 1086). The **source of the River**

Test, at first screened by waterside willows and poplars, lies in a large pool over in the field to the right, on private land, but this special place can be contemplated and enjoyed over or through the hawthorn hedge by the track. At the end of the lime avenue, turn briefly **left** to join the **farm track** then **RIGHT** to take you along the lane to Holy Trinity Church (V) on the corner, and into the tranquil Medieval settlement of **Ashe.** At the **T-junction** turn **RIGHT** for a short distance along the quiet country lane to Ashe House (VI) on your right, a beautifully-proportioned Georgian house, with a fanlight over the door, a walled garden and an orchard with apple blossom in season.

(4) Having enjoyed the Jane Austen associations here, **retrace your steps** back towards Overton, across the water meadow by the stream to **(2)** on the map. **At (2) go through the gate and turn RIGHT** for approx **100m** at the foot of the sloping field, then **RIGHT** again to follow a short green lane over a couple of footbridges, enabling the walker to cross the ford. At a No Through Road turn **LEFT** by Polhampton Farmhouse (VII) to head back westwards in the direction of Overton, along a quiet road. Note that the river, a mere trickle a short while ago, is now a broad, peaceful, watery expanse.

(5) Immediately before **Coney Field House** on the right, with its distinctive chimneys and thick box hedge, leave the country lane and turn **RIGHT** up a

green byway which leads to the **minor road** heading NE from Overton towards Ashe Warren.

(6) When you reach the road, turn **RIGHT** to follow it over a chalk ridge and down to a **crossroads**.

(7) At the crossroads turn **LEFT** to head NW along another quiet country road. This is the **Harrow Way,** lined with oaks along its NE side, and will be followed for some distance.

(8) After approx **400m**, where the modern road branches off to the right, continue **STRAIGHT AHEAD** along a **byway open to all traffic** – the Harrow Way – as it slowly gains height. You are now on the old drove road (VIII), following in the footsteps of those 18[th]century shepherds herding their flocks along this ancient ridgeway. In due course, gaps in the hedge on your right may offer glimpses of the rolling down-land of North Hampshire, with the line of the Portway Roman Road (see Walk 5) just visible on the northern horizon, marked by a jagged line of conifers.

(9) Cross the **B3051** Overton-Kingsclere road **WITH GREAT CARE**, away from the corner, and continue **AHEAD** along the **Harrow Way**, a byway open to all traffic. Here this ancient track leads through a broad belt of deciduous woodland, with thickets of hawthorn, hazel (magnificent catkins in February), elder, ivy and gnarled old fruit trees, laced with sprawling wild clematis. Approx **500m**

after crossing the Kingsclere road, keep an eye open for a footpath crossing the **Harrow Way**, to help locate your position, but **carry on past this** and continue along the Harrow Way. Trees are taller here – centuries-old beeches and oaks with pendulous creepers. You are following in ancient steps, going back over 4000 years.

(10) After **a further approx 400m** (ie just under 1km beyond the B3051) at grid ref **SU505 515**, watch for tracks from right and left crossing the Harrow Way. On the left there is **a wooden signpost with a red arrow tacked on halfway down.** Concrete barriers may be in position, and there are two No Entry road signs for cars Nov-May. **Turn LEFT here** to leave the Harrow Way and head southwards **back towards Overton** along **Court Drove**, perhaps imagining the shepherds heading down to market (see 'Imagine the Scene'). This is appropriately named **Court** Drove for a reason that will become clear shortly. After crossing the railway bridge, you will come to the Junior School on your right. Over in the fields on your left lies the site of the Medieval Deer Park. Follow the village road down to the bend, where **Silk Mill Lane** joins from the right. Along here once stood the **first water-powered silk mill in Southern England**, built in 1769, demolished in 1848, where raw imported silk was converted into thread for the Spitalfields silk weavers. Carry on round the bend to the left, **down the hill**, to bring you past Court Farmhouse (IX) on your left, and,

138

shortly, to the Church of St Mary.   Medieval, with later alterations, it is suggested that the original tower arch and west bay of the nave were rebuilt c1588 using monastic stone, possibly from Titchfield Abbey.

(11)Beyond the church, at the **T-junction**, turn **RIGHT** to take you back down Kingsclere Road to the traffic lights at the crossroads in the centre of the village, where the White Hart (X) forms a fitting end to this Post-Medieval walk.   Whilst enjoying some well-deserved refreshment here, and having admired the Tudor Rose emblem above the grand stone fireplace in the front room, you might like to imagine the excitement and commotion of one November night in 1805, when Lt. John Lapenotiere, Captain of HMS 'Pickle', burst in with news of victory in the Battle of Trafalgar, but sadly the death of Lord Nelson. The Trafalgar Way plaque near the Community Centre across the road gives further details.
On leaving the White Hart, take a moment to look across the road to wide Winchester Street, lined with 15th-19thcentury historic buildings, where the annual sheep fair once took place. Complete the short distance back up London Road towards Basingstoke, and the car park at Turnpike Cottages.

HISTORICAL and ARCHAEOLOGICAL NOTES
(multi-period)

A visit to the Willis Museum, Basingstoke, is highly recommended.

(I) Overton: a charter of AD909 refers to *Uferantun* ('Higher Farmstead') being granted by King Edward the Elder to Frithstan, Bishop of Winchester. The Manor of Overton remained in episcopal hands until 1869, apart from during the Commonwealth (1649-60). Domesday (1086) records that the village had four mills and two churches, one of which is referred to as a 'Superior Church', a term usually reserved for a minster. In the early 13th century the Bishop of Winchester established seven new market towns across Hampshire to increase revenue, one of which was Overton.

(II) Turnpikes: Turnpike Trusts were set up in the 18th century to raise money for road repairs by charging tolls. Previously, maintenance had been in the hands of parishes, and many roads were in a shocking state of disrepair. The Andover and Basingstoke Turnpike was opened in 1754.

(III) Overton Mill, formerly Portals Paper Mill: paper-making developed in the area in the early 18th century when Henry Portal, a Huguenot, took over the lease of Bere Mill on the Test (see Walk 6 Note IX) and began producing paper for the Bank of England. Overton Mill still makes banknotes for the B. of E. and other countries. Jane Austen and her family were acquainted with the Portals, and two of her brother Edward's sons went on to marry members of the Portal family.

(IV) Mesolithic flint blade (BC10000-4001) found next to the footpath.

(V) Holy Trinity Church, Ashe: 19[th]century but on the site of an older building. A late 13[th]century coin found in the mortar suggests that the old church dated from this time, though the discovery of a Norman *piscina* (stone basin) built into one of the walls implies an earlier origin.

(VI) Ashe House (late 18th/early 19[th]century): it was here that a high-spirited young Jane Austen flirted with Tom Lefroy, nephew of her close friend who lived there. A proposal was expected, but after an evening spent together in the garden (behind the yew hedge to the right of the house), Tom left abruptly for Ireland, and the dalliance was at an end. Was Jane's fortune perhaps not substantial enough?

(VII) Polhampton and Polhampton Farmhouse: first documented in AD940, *Polemetune* is mentioned in Domesday as having two mills and a church. Though a church dating to pre-1066, and its replacement built in c1340, are known to have existed, the exact location of these is not confirmed. Polhampton Farmhouse dates to the mid-17[th]century. Approx 500m to the east of Polhampton Farmhouse, 20 pieces of **Neolithic flint** (BC4000-2201) were found, including several axes, one of which was polished. A leaf-shaped arrowhead and 12 scrapers were seen in the Willis

Museum in 1956, where a good display of flint scrapers from other sites can be viewed.

(VIII) Old drove road: although droving reached its peak in the 18th/19[th]century, it was well-established by the Middle Ages, with prehistoric origins. When the central track became over-used, a parallel track often formed over the years, as here.

(IX) Court Farmhouse is an open hall house, tree-ring dated to 1496-1505, which served as an early episcopal palace for the Bishop of Winchester, as well as a courthouse where the manorial court took place, under the aegis of the Bishop's steward.

(X) White Hart Inn: although the origins of the White Hart date to the Middle Ages (a Latin document of 1442 refers to a *hospitium*, inn, on the site), the glory days of this old coaching inn came in the 18[th]century. At least 70 scheduled coaches, carrying mail and passengers along the Great Western Road from London to Exeter, arrived each week, at all hours of the day and night. Food, drink and replacement horses had to be provided – within the space of 20minutes! The coming of the railways in the 19[th]century marked the end of coaching inns, but the White Hart continued to survive as a village inn, much as it does today. **Town Mill**, now residential, lies behind the White Hart car park. A watermill existed here in 1728, possibly earlier, before being rebuilt as a corn mill in the 19[th]century, and later used as a pulp mill to supply Laverstoke Paper Mill until the early 1920s.

Palaeolithic BC500,000-10001 Mesolithic 10000-4001	Neolithic BC4000-2201	Bronze Age BC2200-801	Iron Age BC800-AD42

Roman AD43-409	Early Med/Saxon AD410-1065	Medieval AD1066-1539	Post-Med AD1540-1900

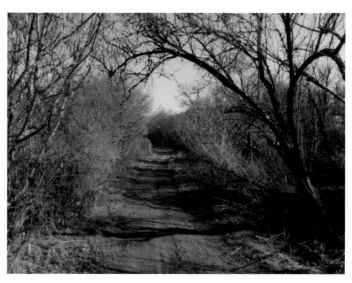

*Harrow Way between **(9)** and **(10)***

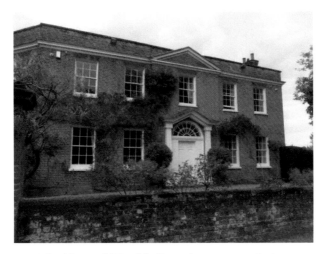

Ashe House (VI) with Jane Austen associations

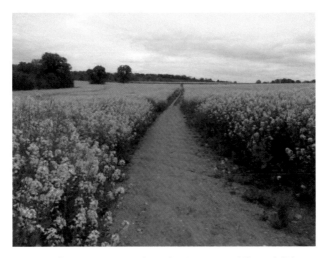

Heading east towards Ashe between (1) and (2)

EPILOGUE: A LINEAR WALK (OS Explorer 144)

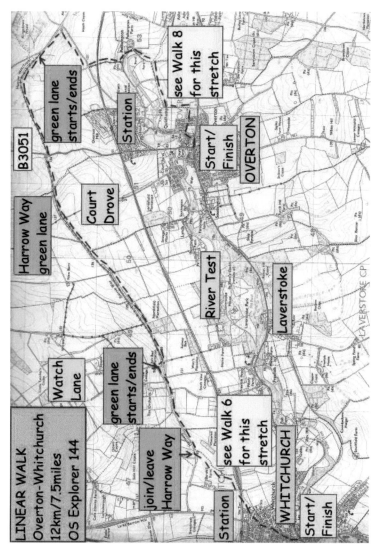

EPILOGUE: LINEAR WALK: A Final Experience

**Approx distance: 12-13km/7.5-8.1miles.
Challenging.
Refreshments/Toilets:** Tea rooms and pubs in Whitchurch and Overton. Public toilets in Whitchurch, Bell Street car park.

This linear route forms a fitting conclusion to the 'Harrow Way Experience', covering the best-preserved stretch of green lane between **Overton** and **Whitchurch**, accessible by public transport:
**Stagecoach Bus 76, Andover-Basingstoke
South West Trains, stations at start and finish.**

The walk can be followed in either direction, each offering a different historical experience:
Whitchurch-Overton (W-E) provides a **'Medieval Experience'**, following the route taken by **shepherds and drovers** in the Middle Ages, herding their flocks and cattle to the markets of Overton and London.
Overton-Whitchurch (E-W) provides a **'Bronze Age Experience'**, walking westwards with those coppersmiths and traders in pursuit of Cornwall's tin, or early pilgrims making their way along the *hearg weg* ('way to the shrine or holy place') towards the ritual centres of Salisbury Plain.

To give the walk a focus, keep an eye open for:
> Drove road indicators: terrace of up to 20m in width, with a narrow tarmac strip/unsurfaced track flanked by grassy verges, bounded by banks

or hedges to funnel flocks. Sometimes a parallel track has been created, over time, still within the boundary banks, where the original route has become too worn.

> **Ridgeway or terrace-way:** does the trackway run along the crest of the ridge? Or offset, on a terrace below the ridge? Or neither?

> **Bronze Age tree species:** how many species familiar to Bronze Age travellers still line the ancient trackway? After the ice sheets retreated, birch, aspen and sallow (low willow) began to spread northwards from around BC10000, colonising the tundra and moorland; pine and hazel followed from cBC8500, with oak, alder, lime, elm, holly, ash, beech, hornbeam and maple arriving in succession.

Nature lovers and history lovers alike will find much to enjoy and reflect upon during this exhilarating walk, whatever the season – autumn colours, spring greenery, summer shadows, winter winds. Perhaps, though, it is important to let the present gradually slip away, and take a step back into older time, for your final experience of walking the Harrow Way through the Ages.

To complement your 'Harrow Way Experience', why not visit the museums and places of interest listed on page 164?

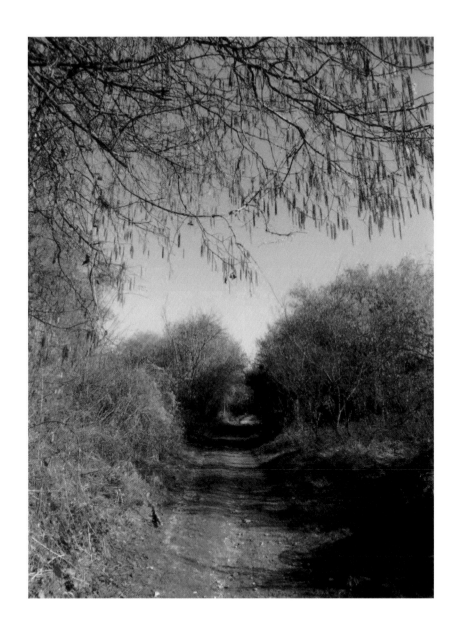

GLOSSARY

AGGER: substantial raised surface of Roman road.
Walk 5

ARD: simple plough, drawn by oxen, dating from the Neolithic.
Walk 4

BANJO ENCLOSURES: oval or circular enclosures surrounded by a ditch and bank, approached by a long, funnel-shaped avenue, up to 90m in length, which may have served a corall function. Probably associated with farming/stock-rearing practices, some have also revealed evidence of settlement. Often found near other enclosures, field systems and trackways, they date mainly from the Middle Iron Age (BC300-101). Found principally in Wessex.
Walk 4

BARROWS or BURIAL MOUNDS:
Neolithic long barrows: communal burial mounds, containing the remains, often disarticulated, of men, women and children.
Walk 2

Bronze Age barrows: funerary monuments containing single or, sometimes, multiple burials or cremations, the latter more common after BC2000. Though roughly circular, there were variations on the basic shape, including bowl, disc and bell barrows. **Bowl barrows** (cBC2400-1500), the most numerous, were sometimes ditched, covering single or multiple burials, constructed of earth or rubble. They occur either in isolation, or grouped as cemeteries. **Disc barrows** (cBC1600-1200) have a

149

lower profile, consisting of a central platform, sometimes raised above the surrounding land, with an outer bank and ditch. Small mounds on the disc cover the burials. Not common, disc barrows occur mainly in Wessex.
Walks 3 & 5

BEAKER PERIOD: transitional period between Neolithic and Bronze Age, cBC2500-2200. Migrants from Central Europe, probably originating in the Eurasian Steppes, brought metalworking skills, new burial practices and distinctive pottery, including the inverted bell-shaped drinking vessel which gives the culture its name (good examples in the museums in Andover, Basingstoke & Salisbury).
Walk 3

BURGAGE: Medieval land term, a burgage was a town 'rental property', owned by king or lord, consisting of a house on a long, thin plot of land, with a narrow street frontage.
Walk 6

'CELTIC' FIELD SYSTEMS: not related to Celtic culture, these early agricultural field systems date from any time in the Early Bronze Age (BC2200-1601) to the Early Medieval period (AD411-1065).
Walk 4

CIST: prehistoric stone-lined coffin, containing a body or cremated remains.
Walk 5

CROPMARKS/PARCHMARKS: patterns in the growth of crops or grass that show up in aerial photos, giving indications of what lies beneath the soil surface, and which may not be visible from the ground. Underlying ditches, walls and compacted surfaces cause subtle variations in colour and growth of crops.

All walks

DEMESNE: land worked by peasants for the lord of the manor's profit.

Walk 7

DESERTED MEDIEVAL SETTLEMENT/VILLAGE (DMS/DMV): a former settlement, abandoned during the Middle Ages, typically leaving no trace except for 'lumps and bumps' or cropmarks. Whilst reasons for desertion may have included environmental changes, or the effects of the Black Death in the 14th century, the majority of settlements seem to have been abandoned during the 15th century, when landowners took advantage of the profitable wool trade to turn arable land into pasture, or to enclose arable land. In the Post-Medieval period, the fashion for landscaped parkland accounted for the removal of 'eyesore' villages and their occupants. Note that a **Deserted** Medieval Settlement or Village refers to a settlement with fewer than three inhabited dwellings; a **Shrunken** Medieval Village is where there are more than three inhabited dwellings.

Walks 2, 3 & 7

DOMESDAY BOOK: a comprehensive survey, commissioned by William I in 1086, to assess the full extent of the wealth and manpower of his newly-conquered kingdom.

Walk 7, and villages mentioned in other walks

151

DROVE ROADS: trackways used by shepherds and drovers to herd animals from country to town, from one area to another, or in search of pasture. Also known as 'driftways' or 'green roads', they may well have been in use since prehistoric times.
Walks 2, 3, 4, 6, 7, 8 & linear route

FULLING: process in wool production involving cleansing and beating the cloth, to help fibres knit.
Walk 6

HIDE: amount of land necessary to sustain a peasant household.
Walk 7

HENGE: prehistoric ceremonial enclosure.
Walks 2 & 3

HUNDRED: subdivision of the shire based on groups of estates totalling 100 hides (see above).
Walk 6

INTAGLIOS: similar to signet rings, used by the rich and powerful in Roman times to stamp documents by pressing the ring into hot wax.
Walk 5

ISOTOPIC ANALYSIS: scientific method used to reconstruct past environmental and climatic conditions, to investigate human and animal diets in the past. Isotope analysis of enamel on teeth can tell us where/how a person lived.
Walks 2 & 3

LYNCHETS: evidence of early ploughing (Early Bronze Age – Early Medieval).
Walk 1

MANOR: an estate with land, and jurisdiction over tenants. Not necessarily a whole village, which might have several manors, just as one manor might own land in more than one village.

Walk 7

MANORIAL COURT: Medieval manorial courts were held on average every three weeks. They were presided over by the lord of the manor himself, or his steward, with jurors elected by the villagers, and all serfs (agricultural workers) were obliged to attend. Issues such as land boundaries and grazing rights were settled, as well as disputes relating to, for example, non-repayment of loans, theft, and selling ale before it was approved by the ale taster. Courts took place either in the manor house itself, the church nave, or the open air.

Walks 7 & 8

NEOLITHIC POTTERY:

Fengate ware: a sub-style of Peterborough ware, dating to the Middle Neolithic (BC3500-3000/2800).

Grooved ware: dates to the Later Neolithic/Early Bronze Age (BC3200-1800).

Walk 6

OPUS SIGNINUM: building material for pavements in Roman houses, consisting of tiles broken up into very small pieces, mixed with mortar then beaten down. A technique inherited from the Phoenicians, it was popular from the 1stcentury BC to about the 2ndcentury AD.

Walk 2

PALSTAVE: a type of Bronze Age axe, with a more sophisticated method of attaching the handle than its precursor, the simple flat axe.   Walk 5

REEVE: in Anglo-Saxon times, a local official, in particular the chief magistrate of a town or district. Post-Conquest, the term denoted the lord of the manor's official, who supervised labour dues and renders owed by peasants.
Walk 6

RING DITCH: form of earthwork which may have surrounded round barrows or roundhouses.
Walk 3

ROMAN/ROMANO-BRITISH POTTERY:
Alice Holt/Farnham ware: grey kitchenware, sometimes with combing or white paint.

Black-burnished ware: a type of Romano-British ceramic.

New Forest ware: in the 3rdcentury AD, favourable conditions led to the New Forest becoming an important centre of pottery production, including both fine tableware and coarse kitchenware. Fabrics ranged from buff to grey.

Oxfordshire ware: this included Late Imitation Samian, with a pink-orange fabric, and Parchment ware, with a fine white powdery fabric.

Samian ware: high status red glossy pottery made in the 1st and 2nd centuries AD in South, East and Central Gaul (France and Germany). Some pieces are plain, but many are highly decorated with animals, plants and figures.
Walks 2, 3 & 5

SHRUNKEN MEDIEVAL VILLAGE: see 'Deserted Medieval Village' p151.

154

SUNKEN-FEATURED BUILDING (SFB): term used in Early Medieval architecture for a small to medium-sized timber building with sunken floor. A tradition in N Europe, spanning 5th-11thcenturies AD, with much older origins.
Walk 3

'THAMES PICKS': see 'tranchet axes' below.

THEGNS: Pre-Conquest nobles below the level of earls, thegns were local estate owners with at least five hides of land, some owning grand halls. They formed an essential part of the king's army.
Walk 6

TRANCHET AXES (adzes): Mesolithic tools, which continued into the Neolithic, found in abundance in Hampshire, where the flint is of superior quality. They consist of a flint blade hafted into a wooden handle, which rarely survives. Probably used for digging, clearing, tree-felling and woodworking, including making dug-out canoes, they are also known as **'Thames Picks'**, as so many have been dredged from the river. The Willis Museum, Basingstoke, has an extensive collection, George Willis having been a keen 'flinter' in the 1920s, as does Andover Museum of the Iron Age.
Walks 1, 2 & 3

TURNPIKES: Trusts set up in the 18thcentury to raise money for road repairs by charging tolls.
Walk 8

WHITE HART (as a pub name): personal badge of Richard 11 (1367-1400), adopted by innkeepers to show their loyalty.
Walks 3, 6 & 8

REFERENCES and SOURCES

Allen, D; Gould, S; Johnson, L; King, J; with help from **Elliot, S.** *Buried in Time – the Neolithic. Nutbane Longbarrow* (Report published in the Proceedings of the Prehistoric Society, 1959)

Bedoyere de la, G. *Roman Britain: A New History* (Thames and Hudson, 2006)

Channel 4. *Bone Detectives: Britain's Buried Secrets* (25 Jan 2020, Episode 3)

Cochrane, C. *The Lost Roads of Wessex* (Pan Books Ltd, 1969)

Codrington, T. *Roman Roads in Britain* (Society for Promoting Christian Knowledge, 1919)

Coghlan, H H. *The Old Way from Basingstoke to Salisbury Plain.* Transactions of the Newbury District Field Club, Vol 7 (1934-37) pages 151-59 (Historic England Archive)

Coppen, M. *Henry White of Fyfield: A Georgian Parson in his Place* (Maryacre Publishing, 2017)

Cunliffe, B. *Britain Begins* (OUP, 2013)

Edwards, A M. *In the Steps of Jane Austen* (Arcady Books, 1985)

Fasham, P; Whinney, R. *Roads to the Past: A Summary of Recent Archaeological Excavations near Winchester* (Trust for Wessex Archaeology and City of Winchester, 1985)

Flambert, J. *Littleton Farm in the Parish of Kimpton* (Jane Flambert, 2011)

Fort, T. *The A303: Highway to the Sun* (Simon & Schuster UK Ltd, 2012)

Grinsell, L V. *The Archaeology of Wessex* (Methuen, 1958)

Grinsell, L V. *Proceedings of the Hampshire Field Club,* in Hampshire Barrows, Vol 14 (1938) p28, p30

Hampshire Cultural Trust – see O'Malley, M.

Hampshire Historic Environment Record, HCC

Hampshire County Council Collections, Chilcomb House, Winchester (01962 678140)

Hampshire Printing Services. *Exploring Overton. (Proceeds in aid of St Michael's Hospice)*

Henig, M; Soffe, G. *The Thruxton Roman Villa and its Mosaic Pavement.* Journal of the British Archaeological Association, Vol 146, Issue 1 (1993)

Higham, Nicholas J; Ryan, Martin J. *The Anglo-Saxon World* (Yale University Press, New Haven & London, 2015)

Hilts, C. *Writing Early Medieval England* (Current Archaeology 346, Jan 2019)

Hindle, P. *Medieval Roads and Tracks* (Shire Publications, part of Bloomsbury Publishing plc, 2018)

Hippisley Cox, R. *The Green Roads of England* (The Lost Library, Glastonbury, first published by Methuen, 1914)

Hunter, J; Ralston, I (Ed). *The Archaeology of Britain.* Chapter 5, *The Earlier Bronze Age,* Mike Parker Pearson (Routledge, 1999)

Jacques, D; Lyons, T; Phillips, T. *Blick Mead: Exploring the 'first place' in the Stonehenge Landscape* (Current Archaeology 324, March 2017)

Langlands, A. *The Ancient Ways of Wessex* (Windgather Press, Oxbow Books, 2019)

Lewis, C; Harding, P; Aston, M; Tayler, T (Ed). *Time Team's Timechester: A Companion to Archaeology* (Channel 4 Books, 2002)

Margary, I. *Roman Roads in Britain,* Vol 1 (Phoenix House, 1955)

Oliver, J. *The Ancient Roads of England* (Cassell, 1945)

Oliver, N. *A History of Ancient Britain* (BBC dvd, 2011)

O'Malley, M. *When the Mammoth Roamed Romsey: A Study of the Prehistory of Romsey and Devizes* (LTVAS, 1982). Series by David Allen; Gould S; King J; Johnson L; Stone P. Willis Archive held by Hampshire Cultural Trust

Parker Pearson, M. *The Age of Stonehenge.* Paper in Antiquity 81 p267

Parker Pearson, M. *Bronze Age Britain* (English Heritage, London, 2005)

Quarley Church leaflet *Church of St Michael, Quarley*

Stowe, A. *Roman Roving* (Mayfield Press, 2018)

Swan, Vivien G. *Pottery in Roman Britain* (Shire Publications Ltd, 1975)

The Churches Conservation Trust, *The Church of St Nicholas, Freefolk, Hampshire,* series 4, no 77 (revised 1997)

The Deserted Medieval Village Research Group, Annual Reports 18-21 (1970-73) pages 13-14 (Historic England Archive)

Timperley, H W; Brill, E. *Ancient Trackways of Wessex* (The History Press, 2013)

TVBC *Literary Test Valley* (leaflet)

Victoria County History, Hampshire, Vol 4 (1911) p206 and p299 (DMV Research Group)

Waldram, R. *A History of the White Hart at Overton* (2015)

Whittle, J. *Exploring Prehistoric Paths: Twenty Wessex Walks* (The Hobnob Press, 1988)

Winbolt, S E. *Roman Sites on the Harrow Way in the Basingstoke Area.* Papers and Proceedings of the HFC&AS, Vol 15 (1941) page 245 (Historic England Archive)

Wood, M. *King Alfred and the Anglo-Saxons* (BBC, August 2013)

Wood, M. *The Domesday Quest: In Search of the Roots of England* (BBC Books, 2005)

Wymer, J J; Bonsall, C (Ed) *Gazetteer of Mesolithic Sites in England and Wales* (1977)

Lecture and Seminar Notes

Allen, D. Curator of Hampshire Archaeology for the Hampshire Cultural Trust. *Building, Growing, Milling and Brewing: Roman Ways on the Hampshire Chalk.* Annual conference of the Hampshire Field Club and Archaeological Society, 5 Nov 2016

Clutterbuck, J. Project Manager, Cotswold Archaeology. *Excavations at Aldi Execution Site.* Lecture at Andover Museum, 5 April 2015

Pollard, J. Professor of Archaeology, Univ of Southampton. *Latest Research on the Neolithic/ Early Bronze Age Transition.* Annual conference of the HFC&AS, 17 Nov 2018

Websites
www.ancientcraft.co.uk
www.aprilmunday.wordpress.com
www.archaeologydataservice.ac.uk
www.archive.org
www.asprom.org
www.brendaparkerway.northhampshiredownsramblers.org.uk
www.british-history.ac.uk
www.britishlistedbuildings.co.uk
www.conservationhandbooks.com
www.english-heritage.org.uk
www.fairgroundcraft.co.uk
www.hampshirearchaeology.wordpress.com
www.hampshireculture.org.uk
www.hampshire-history.com
www.hantsfieldclub.org.uk
www.hants.gov.uk
www.localdroveroads.co.uk
www.pentonmewsey.org.uk
www.research.hgt.org.uk
www.telegraph.co.uk
www.victoriacountyhistory.ac.uk
www.visit-hampshire.co.uk
www.wikipedia.org.com
www.winchester-cathedral.org.uk

Maps
OS Mapping © Crown Copyright 2021 Licence 100059949
Ancient Trackways of Wessex, Timperley, HW & Brill, E, by kind permission of The History Press (2013)

THANKS and ACKNOWLEDGEMENTS

A-HARROWING *We Shall Go* (thanks to Neville and Anne for the inspired title) would not have seen the light of day without the help and support of the following:

David Hopkins, Hampshire County Archaeologist, and Alan Whitney, Historic Data Manager, HCC, both of whom gave guidance, encouragement and initial inspiration for this venture, with Alan kindly providing data from the Historic Environment Record.

My grateful thanks go to all the following: Danny Crane-Brewer and the staff of Mayfield Press; Ross Turle, Curatorial Liaison Manager, Hampshire Cultural Trust, for information about Hampshire County Council Collections, permission to use the photos on p30 and p163, and the artist's impression of the construction of Nutbane Long Barrow p45; the artist Mike Codd; Gareth Swain and Anette Fuhrmeister at The History Press for permission to use maps from Timperley and Brill's *Ancient Trackways of Wessex*; Ordnance Survey; David Hopkins, in a private capacity, for his delightful line drawings; the Manager, staff and volunteers at Andover Museum/Museum of the Iron Age, for their enthusiastic support of my projects; the Directors, staff and volunteers of Butser Ancient Farm; the Venue Manager, staff and volunteers at the Willis Museum and Sainsbury Gallery, Basingstoke; staff at the Wiltshire and Swindon History Centre, and at local museums including

Salisbury, Reading, West Berkshire and Winchester, all of whom have been helpful in providing information; Cynthia Poole, Director of Quarley Down Ancient Environs Project, for her patience and knowledge; Dave Allen for his useful pointers and suggestions; Richard Donovan for his technical expertise; Gill Baker for information on St Nicholas' Church, and John Isherwood on Nutbane Long Barrow excavation.

For the piloting of walks I am indebted to modern-day Harrow Wayfarers John R and Mandy, John B and Tim, Anita and Gordon, Sue and Mike, Louise and Huw, Hilary and friends.

For proof-reading (and sharing the fun of our literary projects) I am extremely grateful to Anne, for her patience and care. Any remaining mistakes are mine, for which I apologise.

To my family I owe a debt of gratitude: to Miriam for her experienced eye and pertinent suggestions, and Chloe for helpful comments and observations; to Jo and Roland for ongoing interest; to the professional archaeologists Neville and Chris for keeping an 'enthusiastic amateur' on track; to all patient friends who have supported me throughout.

A special thank you to Neville for his professional advice, encouragement - and the occasional gentle prod!

And finally ... thanks to the Harrow Way itself for giving me such an absorbing project during lockdown.   April 2021

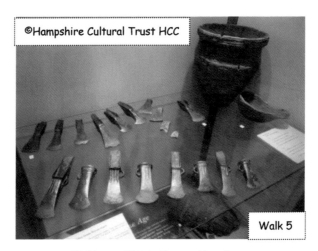

Walk 5

Cholderton Estate Bronze Hoard
Foreground: four palstaves and four socketed axes
Rear right: collared urn, cremation and pottery scoop
Andover Museum of the Iron Age

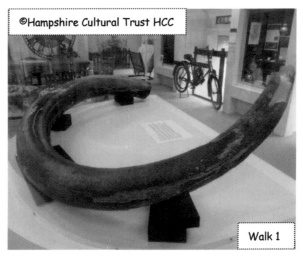

Walk 1

20,000 year old woolly mammoth tusk, 2.8m end to tip
The Willis Museum, Basingstoke

163

MUSEUMS and PLACES TO VISIT
Museums and Centres mentioned in this Guide:
Andover Museum and Museum of the Iron Age
Willis Museum and Sainsbury Gallery, Basingstoke
Butser Ancient Farm, Chalton, Waterlooville
Amesbury History Centre
The Salisbury Museum
West Berkshire Museum, Newbury
Reading Museum
Whitchurch Silk Mill
Winchester City Museum

Further visits for history- and nature lovers:
Basing House
Curtis Museum, Alton
Eastleigh Museum
East Meon Sustainability Centre
Gilbert White's House and Gardens, Selborne
Jane Austen's House and Museum, Chawton
King John's House and Museum, Romsey
Milestones Museum, Basingstoke
Old Sarum
Petersfield Museum
Queen Elizabeth Country Park
Silchester Roman Walls and Amphitheatre
Westgate Museum, Winchester
Wiltshire Museum, Devizes

Visits can be arranged by appointment to:
Hampshire County Council Collections,
Chilcomb House, Winchester (01962 678140)
www.hampshireculture.org.uk

Modern-Day Harrow Wayfarers ...

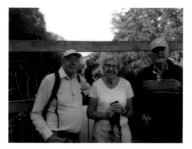

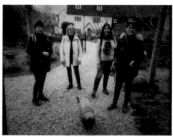

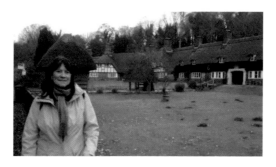

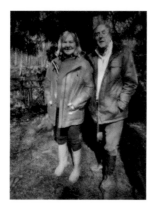

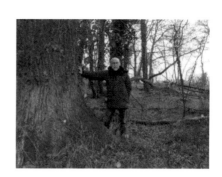

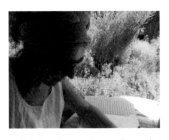

At work in the garden
Following in the tradition of *Roman Roving* (2018), *A-Harrowing We Shall Go* is aimed at encouraging ramblers and 'armchair ramblers' to explore the historic and archaeological landscape that lies all around them.

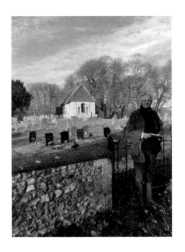

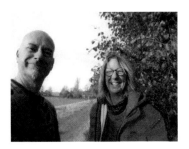

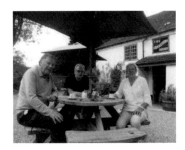

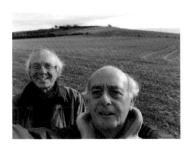